A prescription Guide for Metoprolol Tartrate

Understanding Its Role in Managing Hypertension, Angina, and Heart Failure

Dr. Thane Mercer

Copyright © 2025 Dr. Thane Mercer
All rights reserved.
No part of this publication may be reproduced, distributed, or transmitted in any form or by any means, including photocopying, recording, or other electronic or mechanical methods, without the prior written permission of the publisher, except in the case of brief quotations embodied in critical reviews and certain other noncommercial uses permitted by copyright law

DISCLAIMER

This book, Metoprolol Tartrate: Comprehensive Insights into Usage, Safety, and Efficacy, is intended for informational purposes only and does not replace professional medical advice, diagnosis, or treatment. The information provided in this book is based on existing knowledge and research available at the time of writing. Every effort has been made to ensure accuracy, but the content may not reflect the most current developments in medicine.

Readers are advised to consult qualified healthcare professionals for specific medical advice and to address any questions or concerns related to the use of Metoprolol Tartrate or other medical conditions. This book is not a substitute for personalized care from licensed physicians, pharmacists, or other healthcare providers.

The author and publisher assume no liability for any risks or damages arising directly or indirectly from the use or application of the information contained in this book. Always follow the guidance of your healthcare provider and adhere to prescribed medical regimens.

This book is not intended to promote or endorse any specific medication, treatment, or therapy. The mention of Metoprolol Tartrate or any other medication is for educational purposes and should not be interpreted as a recommendation or endorsement.

For any medical emergencies, seek immediate assistance from a licensed healthcare provider or emergency services.

"**An Invaluable Resource for Medical Professionals and Patients Alike**"

Metoprolol Tartrate: Comprehensive Insights into Usage, Safety, and Efficacy by Dr. Thane Mercer is a remarkable guide that offers both depth and clarity. The book excels in breaking down complex medical concepts into accessible language without sacrificing scientific accuracy. It's a must-read for anyone looking to understand this vital medication.

Dr. Amanda Keller, Cardiologist

"**An Expertly Crafted and Informative Guide**"

Dr. Thane Mercer delivers an exceptionally detailed and engaging exploration of Metoprolol Tartrate. Her expertise shines through every chapter, making this book a go-to reference for healthcare providers and an empowering resource for patients managing heart-related conditions.

Dr. Thomas Nguyen, Clinical Pharmacologist

"A Comprehensive and Reader-Friendly Book"

This book blends professional knowledge with accessible writing, making it perfect for both the medical community and lay readers. Dr. Thane Mercer's attention to detail ensures readers gain a thorough understanding of Metoprolol Tartrate, its uses, and its safety.

Samantha Reed, Registered Nurse

"**Essential Reading for Understanding Beta-Blockers**"

Dr. Thane Mercer provides an authoritative and compassionate look into Metoprolol Tartrate. Her thoughtful approach demystifies the medication and equips readers with the knowledge to approach their treatment with confidence.

Dr. Kevin Simmons, Pharmacology Professor

"A Masterpiece in Medical Literature"

This book is a testament to Dr. Thane Mercer's dedication to improving patient education. It's comprehensive, informative, and an indispensable guide for understanding the intricacies of Metoprolol Tartrate.

Dr. Elise Morgan, Internal Medicine Specialist

TABLE OF CONTENTS

TABLE OF CONTENTS	**10**
INTRODUCTION	**12**
CHAPTER ONE	**28**
What Is Metoprolol Tartrate?	28
Why Understanding the Difference Matters	33
CHAPTER TWO	**41**
Metoprolol Tartrate's Mode of Action	41
How Metoprolol Tartrate Works	43
Pharmacokinetics of Metoprolol Tartrate	48
Dosage Forms of Metoprolol Tartrate	57
CHAPTER THREE	**64**
Primary Indications of Metoprolol Tartrate	64
Off-Label Uses of Metoprolol Tartrate	73
CHAPTER FOUR: Administration and Dosage	**82**
Guidelines for Use of Metoprolol Tartrate	82
Special Populations and Metoprolol Tartrate	92
Drug Interactions with Metoprolol Tartrate	104
CHAPTER FIVE: Side Effects and Risks	**117**
Common Side Effects of Metoprolol Tartrate	117
Severe Risks of Metoprolol Tartrate	121
Warnings and Precautions for Metoprolol Tartrate	127
Handling Overdose of Metoprolol Tartrate	135
CHAPTER SIX: Comparative Analysis	**142**
Metoprolol vs. Other Beta-Blockers	142

CHAPTER SEVEN. Patient Perspectives   **156**
    Case Studies: Real-Life Examples of Patients Benefiting from Metoprolol Tartrate   156

CHAPTER EIGHT: PRACTICAL TIPS FOR PATIENTS   **176**
    How to Manage Side Effects of Metoprolol Tartrate   176

CHAPTER NINE: RESEARCH AND INNOVATIONS   **199**
    Future Potential of Metoprolol Tartrate   210

CHAPTER TEN: FAQs and Myths   **222**

CONCLUSION   **232**

GLOSSARY   **239**

APPENDIX   **249**

INTRODUCTION

Did you know that Metoprolol Tartrate is prescribed to millions of people worldwide every day, acting as a guardian for their hearts? This single, unassuming pill holds the power to slow down a racing heartbeat, lower dangerously high blood pressure, and even prevent the devastating consequences of heart attacks.

The human heart is an extraordinary machine, beating around 100,000 times a day to pump life-sustaining blood through our bodies. Yet, for many people, this miraculous process is threatened by conditions like hypertension, arrhythmias, or the lingering effects of a heart attack. For them, the simple act of living can feel like walking a tightrope. Enter Metoprolol Tartrate, a medication that offers stability, hope, and the chance to reclaim a normal life.

Take the story of Anna, a 45-year-old schoolteacher. Anna had always been full of energy, but after experiencing persistent palpitations, she was diagnosed with tachycardia a condition where her heart raced uncontrollably. Everyday activities like climbing stairs or even reading to her students left her short of breath and exhausted. Her doctor prescribed Metoprolol Tartrate, explaining how it would help regulate her heart rate. Within weeks, Anna's energy returned, and so did her confidence. Today, she enjoys life without the constant fear of her heart racing out of control.

Metoprolol tartrate is a member of the beta-blocker drug class, which is essential to contemporary cardiology. By blocking specific receptors in the heart and blood vessels, it reduces the effects of stress hormones like adrenaline, slowing the heart rate and lowering blood pressure. These effects are lifesaving for patients with conditions such as coronary artery disease, heart failure, or even migraines.

Consider the numbers: over 1 billion people globally suffer from high blood pressure, a leading cause of heart disease and stroke. Medications like

Metoprolol Tartrate play a critical role in reducing these risks, improving not only the quantity but also the quality of life for countless individuals. What makes this drug even more fascinating is its versatility it's not just for high blood pressure. From preventing migraines to treating symptoms of anxiety, Metoprolol Tartrate has become an indispensable tool in the hands of physicians.

But how did this life-saving medication come to be? Who first discovered its potential, and how has it evolved over the years to become a staple in healthcare systems worldwide? What are the mechanisms behind its ability to protect the heart?

In this book, we'll dive deep into the science, history, and human stories that make Metoprolol Tartrate such a remarkable drug. We'll explore its development, how it works at the cellular level, and the profound impact it has had on lives around the world. Whether you're a healthcare professional seeking a deeper understanding, a patient curious about the medication you're taking, or someone intrigued by the marvels of modern medicine, this journey into the heart of Metoprolol Tartrate will be as enlightening as it is inspiring.

Metoprolol Tartrate isn't just a medication it's a symbol of hope and resilience for millions. So, let's begin by uncovering the story of this extraordinary drug and the role it plays in protecting the most vital organ of all: the human heart.

Purpose of the Book: Empowering Readers Through Knowledge

Why write a book about Metoprolol Tartrate? At first glance, it may seem like just another medication among countless others. However, for millions of people worldwide, this tiny pill holds the key to a healthier, longer, and more active life. Whether you're a patient prescribed Metoprolol Tartrate, a caregiver supporting a loved one, or a healthcare professional seeking deeper insights, this book is designed to offer you a comprehensive understanding of this remarkable medication.

Metoprolol Tartrate is more than a beta-blocker; it's a lifeline for people managing heart conditions like hypertension, arrhythmias, and heart failure. It's also used for other conditions, such as preventing migraines and managing symptoms of anxiety. But beyond its medical applications, what makes this drug so essential is the peace of mind it brings to those who rely on it. This book aims to demystify Metoprolol Tartrate its origins, mechanisms, benefits, and risks so that readers can make informed decisions about their health.

Why This Book Matters
For Patients
Taking a new medication can feel overwhelming. Questions often arise: How does this work in my body? What side effects should I expect? Is Is taking it with other drugs safe?* By providing clear, accessible information, this book aims to empower patients. When you understand how Metoprolol Tartrate works, why it's prescribed, and what to

expect, you can feel more in control of your health journey.

For Caregivers

Supporting someone with heart issues can be both rewarding and challenging. Caregivers often play a crucial role in ensuring medications are taken properly and monitoring for potential side effects. This guide will help caregivers feel more confident in their role, offering practical tips and insights to ensure the best outcomes for their loved ones.

For Healthcare Professionals

Whether you're a medical student, nurse, or practicing doctor, this book provides a deep dive into Metoprolol Tartrate's pharmacology, clinical uses, and patient management strategies. It's a practical resource that bridges the gap between scientific knowledge and real-world application.

What You'll Learn

1. The Science Behind Metoprolol Tartrate
- Explore how this medication works at a cellular level to regulate the heart's rhythm and reduce blood pressure.
- Understand its classification as a beta-blocker and what makes it unique compared to other medications in its class.

2. The Human Stories
- Real-life accounts of individuals whose lives have been transformed by Metoprolol Tartrate.
- Insights into the challenges and triumphs of managing chronic heart conditions.

3. The Benefits and Risks
- A balanced view of Metoprolol Tartrate's advantages and potential side effects.
- Guidance on how to recognize and manage common issues, like fatigue or dizziness, and what to do in case of more serious reactions.

4. Practical Advice for Patients and Caregivers

- Tips on taking the medication correctly, including timing, dosage adjustments, and avoiding interactions with certain foods or drugs.
- Advice on lifestyle changes that complement the medication's effects, such as dietary modifications, exercise, and stress management.

5. Beyond the Basics

- Insights into the drug's history: how it was developed, its impact on the field of cardiology, and its evolving role in modern medicine.
- conversations about individualized medicine and beta-blockers' future.

Why This Book Is Unique

Unlike technical medical literature or overly simplistic drug information sheets, this book strikes a balance: it's scientifically rigorous yet easy to understand. It's also comprehensive, offering a full 360-degree view of Metoprolol Tartrate—from its life-saving potential to the realities of living with a chronic condition that necessitates its use.

The Bigger Picture

Ultimately, this book isn't just about Metoprolol Tartrate—it's about understanding the heart and the incredible ways medicine works to protect it. By the end of this guide, readers will have a newfound appreciation for the role this medication plays in safeguarding lives. They'll also gain practical tools to navigate their health journeys with confidence, hope, and clarity.

This book is for you, regardless of your reason for being here. Let's embark on this journey together, learning about the science, stories, and strategies that make Metoprolol Tartrate a cornerstone of modern healthcare.

Why It Matters: The Critical Role of Metoprolol Tartrate in Healthcare

When it comes to healthcare, few medications carry the weight of responsibility that Metoprolol Tartrate does. As a beta-blocker, it serves as a cornerstone in the management of some of the most prevalent and life-threatening conditions, including hypertension, heart attacks, and arrhythmias. Its widespread use underscores its importance, but what makes this medication truly remarkable is the difference it makes in people's lives helping them live longer, healthier, and more fulfilling lives.

A Lifeline for Millions

Cardiovascular illnesses are the main cause of death worldwide, taking millions of lives each year. Conditions like hypertension, arrhythmias, and heart attacks are not just numbers; they represent real people facing daily challenges, from worrying about their next heartbeat to fearing the recurrence of a life-altering cardiac event.

Metoprolol Tartrate steps in as a life-changing ally. By targeting the body's stress response, it slows down the heart rate, reduces blood pressure, and alleviates the strain on the heart. These effects are not merely therapeutic; they are life-saving.

Take hypertension, for example. Known as the "silent killer" because it often shows no symptoms, this condition silently damages arteries and increases the risk of stroke, heart attack, and kidney failure. Metoprolol Tartrate helps to control blood pressure, protecting vital organs from long-term damage and significantly reducing the likelihood of fatal outcomes.

Preventing Heart Attacks

For individuals recovering from a heart attack, Metoprolol Tartrate is nothing short of a miracle drug. After a heart attack, the heart is especially vulnerable to further stress and complications, including another attack. By reducing the workload on the heart and stabilizing its rhythm, Metoprolol Tartrate helps patients recover more safely and prevents future episodes. This makes it a critical component of post-heart-attack care plans, improving survival rates and enhancing quality of life.

Managing Arrhythmias

Arrhythmias irregular heartbeats can range from harmless to life-threatening. For those living with conditions like atrial fibrillation or ventricular tachycardia, the unpredictability of their heart's rhythm can be deeply unsettling. Metoprolol Tartrate works by calming the overactive electrical signals in the heart, restoring a steady and reliable beat. This not only reduces symptoms like dizziness, fatigue, and palpitations but also lowers the risk of severe complications, such as stroke or sudden cardiac arrest.

While its primary focus is on cardiovascular health, Metoprolol Tartrate's versatility extends to other medical uses. It has proven effective in preventing migraines, managing symptoms of hyperthyroidism, and even alleviating anxiety in certain cases. This breadth of application highlights its adaptability and underscores its value in modern medicine.

Bridging the Gap Between Risk and Reward
Every medication carries risks, and Metoprolol Tartrate is no exception. Side effects like fatigue, dizziness, or cold extremities can be challenging, and in rare cases, more serious complicaions can arise. However, its benefits far outweigh these risks for most patients. Healthcare providers carefully assess each individual's needs and tailor treatment plans to ensure the safest and most effective use of the medication.

The key to maximizing its benefits lies in understanding its role. For patients and caregivers, knowing how Metoprolol Tartrate works and why it is prescribed can help alleviate fears and promote better adherence to treatment plans. For healthcare professionals, staying informed about its applications and potential interactions ensures the best outcomes for their patients.

A Pillar of Modern Cardiology

Metoprolol Tartrate is not just a medication; it is a testament to the progress of medical science. Its development marked a significant step forward in the fight against cardiovascular diseases, and its continued use reflects its enduring efficacy and reliability. As a pillar of modern cardiology, it embodies the mission of medicine: to save lives, alleviate suffering, and enhance the human experience.

Why It Matters

In the grand scheme of healthcare, Metoprolol Tartrate is more than just a treatment it's a symbol of hope. For patients grappling with the uncertainties of heart disease, it offers stability. For families, it provides reassurance. For doctors, it's a trusted tool in their arsenal.

This medication matters because it touches lives in profound ways. It allows a grandfather to attend his granddaughter's wedding without worrying about his heart acting up. It gives a young professional the confidence to live fully despite a history of arrhythmias. It offers countless individuals the chance to reclaim their health, one steady heartbeat at a time.

By understanding its role in healthcare, we can better appreciate the transformative impact of Metoprolol Tartrate. Whether you're a patient, caregiver, or medical professional, recognizing why this medication matters deepens our collective commitment to improving lives and underscores the importance of every pill taken, every prescription written, and every life saved.

CHAPTER ONE

What Is Metoprolol Tartrate?

Metoprolol tartrate is a commonly prescribed medicine that is a member of the beta-blocker pharmacological class. It is primarily used to manage cardiovascular conditions such as high blood pressure (hypertension), angina (chest pain), irregular heart rhythms (arrhythmias), and to support recovery and prevention after a heart attack. By reducing the heart's workload and lowering its oxygen demand, Metoprolol Tartrate serves as a critical tool in modern medicine, helping patients achieve better heart health and a higher quality of life.

Definition and Classification

Beta-1 adrenergic receptors are selectively blocked by metoprolol tartrate. This indicates that it targets beta-1 receptors, which are mostly present in the heart. These receptors are responsible for the heart's response to stress hormones like adrenaline. When stimulated, these receptors increase heart rate, blood pressure, and the heart's workload. By blocking these receptors, Metoprolol Tartrate slows the heart rate, decreases blood pressure, and helps the heart pump more efficiently.

Beta-blockers like Metoprolol Tartrate are part of a broader class of medications used to manage cardiovascular conditions. However, Metoprolol's selective nature for beta-1 receptors makes it particularly effective for heart-related conditions with minimal impact on beta-2 receptors, which are found in the lungs and other tissues. This selectivity makes it safer for use in patients with respiratory conditions like asthma, compared to non-selective beta-blockers.

Immediate-Release Formulation
One of the defining features of Metoprolol Tartrate is its immediate-release formulation. This means the medication is designed to be quickly absorbed

into the bloodstream, delivering its effects within a short period. As a result, it often needs to be taken multiple times a day (typically twice) to maintain consistent levels in the body.

Metoprolol Tartrate vs. Metoprolol Succinate: Key Differences

There are two primary types of metoprolol: "Metoprolol Tartrate" and "Metoprolol Succinate". While they share the same active ingredient and belong to the same class of medications, they differ in their formulations, uses, and dosing regimens.

1. Chemical Composition
- Metoprolol. The tartrate salt form of metoprolol is called tartrate, while the succinate salt form is called metoprolol succinate. This difference in chemical composition affects how the drug is released and absorbed in the body.

2. Release Mechanism

- Metoprolol Tartrate is an immediate-release formulation, meaning it is rapidly absorbed and acts quickly but has a shorter duration of effect. Because of this, it is typically given twice or three times a day.
- Metoprolol Succinate, on the other hand, is an extended-release formulation, allowing the drug to be released gradually over time. It only needs to be taken once a day, which can improve convenience and adherence for patients.

3. Primary Uses

- Metoprolol Tartrate is commonly prescribed for acute situations requiring immediate intervention, such as after a heart attack, or for managing symptoms of arrhythmias and angina on a daily basis.
- Metoprolol Succinate is often used for long-term management of chronic

conditions, such as stable heart failure, hypertension, and angina. Its extended-release nature makes it ideal for maintaining consistent blood levels over 24 hours.

4. Dosing

- The dosing regimens differ due to their release mechanisms. Patients taking Metoprolol Tartrate must adhere to more frequent dosing schedules, which can sometimes be challenging. Metoprolol Succinate's once-daily dosing is more convenient but may not be suitable for every condition.

5. Interchangeability

- While both forms of Metoprolol are used for similar conditions, they are not directly interchangeable. A prescription for Metoprolol Tartrate cannot be substituted for Metoprolol Succinate without consulting a healthcare provider, as the differences in release mechanisms and dosing must be carefully considered.

Why Understanding the Difference Matters

The distinction between Metoprolol Tartrate and Metoprolol Succinate is not just a matter of convenience it directly affects treatment outcomes. For example, a patient recovering from a heart attack may benefit from the immediate effects of Metoprolol Tartrate, while someone managing chronic heart failure may achieve better results with the steady, long-lasting effects of Metoprolol Succinate.

A Lifesaving Tool

Understanding what Metoprolol Tartrate is and how it differs from its extended-release counterpart is essential for patients and healthcare providers alike. It ensures that the right medication is chosen for the right condition, optimizing outcomes and improving patients' lives.

Metoprolol Tartrate is more than just a drug it's a lifeline for millions of people around the world. By calming the overworked heart, reducing blood pressure, and preventing dangerous complications, this medication continues to play a pivotal role in the fight against cardiovascular diseases.

Brief History and Development of Metoprolol Tartrate

The story of Metoprolol Tartrate is one of scientific innovation, perseverance, and the relentless pursuit of improving human health. This beta-blocker, now a cornerstone in cardiology, has saved countless lives and transformed the management of cardiovascular diseases. Its journey from concept to widespread use offers a fascinating glimpse into the evolution of modern medicine.

Origins of Beta-Blockers

To understand the history of Metoprolol Tartrate, we must first delve into the broader context of beta-blocker development. Beta-blockers were first conceptualized in the 1950s when researchers began exploring the effects of blocking adrenaline's action on the body. Adrenaline, a key stress hormone, plays a critical role in increasing heart rate, blood pressure, and cardiac workload—actions that are beneficial in emergencies but can be harmful when sustained over time.

The groundwork for beta-blockers was laid by Sir James Black, a Scottish pharmacologist. In 1962, he developed the first beta-blocker, propranolol, which revolutionized the treatment of heart conditions by showing how blocking beta receptors could alleviate angina and control arrhythmias. For his groundbreaking work, Black was awarded the Nobel Prize in Physiology or Medicine in 1988.

The Birth of Metoprolol

Building on the success of propranolol, researchers sought to develop more selective beta-blockers that could target the heart (beta-1 receptors) without significantly affecting other tissues like the lungs (beta-2 receptors). The goal was to reduce side effects, especially for patients with respiratory conditions such as asthma.

In the late 1960s, a team of scientists at the Swedish pharmaceutical company Hässle (now part of AstraZeneca) succeeded in developing Metoprolol. By selectively targeting beta-1 receptors, Metoprolol offered a safer and more effective option for managing heart conditions.

Metoprolol Tartrate, the immediate-release form, was first introduced in the early 1970s. It quickly gained attention for its ability to manage acute and chronic cardiovascular conditions with fewer side effects than earlier beta-blockers. Its rapid absorption and action made it particularly effective for treating sudden cardiac issues, such as angina or post-heart-attack recovery.

Introduction into Medical Practice

Metoprolol Tartrate was officially approved for medical use in 1974, marking the beginning of its journey in clinical practice. Its approval was based on extensive clinical trials demonstrating its efficacy in lowering blood pressure, stabilizing heart rhythms, and reducing the risk of recurrent heart attacks.

Doctors and cardiologists quickly embraced Metoprolol Tartrate for its versatility and effectiveness. It became a go-to treatment for patients recovering from heart attacks, as studies showed it could significantly reduce mortality when administered during and after acute events.

Evolution and Impact

Over the decades, Metoprolol Tartrate has undergone numerous studies, solidifying its reputation as a reliable and essential medication. It became part of standard treatment protocols for a range of conditions, including:

- Hypertension: By controlling blood pressure, it reduces the risk of strokes and heart disease.
- Heart Attack Management: Its ability to decrease heart rate and cardiac stress made it indispensable for improving survival rates.
- Arrhythmias: Metoprolol's role in stabilizing irregular heartbeats has been life-changing for many patients.

In the 1990s, an extended-release version, Metoprolol Succinate, was developed, offering the convenience of once-daily dosing for chronic conditions. While the two forms serve slightly different purposes, both are integral to cardiovascular care.

A Lasting Legacy
Today, Metoprolol Tartrate remains a cornerstone of cardiology. Its development represents a major

milestone in the fight against cardiovascular diseases, and its ongoing use reflects its enduring relevance. The drug's success also paved the way for the development of other selective beta-blockers, further expanding treatment options for patients worldwide.

The Human Impact

Beyond the science and history lies the true significance of Metoprolol Tartrate: the lives it has touched. From patients recovering from heart attacks to those managing chronic hypertension or arrhythmias, this medication has offered hope, stability, and a chance at a healthier future.

The story of Metoprolol Tartrate is a testament to the power of innovation and collaboration in medicine. It stands as a reminder that behind every pill lies a history of scientific discovery and a profound impact on human health.

CHAPTER TWO

Metoprolol Tartrate's Mode of Action

Metoprolol Tartrate's effectiveness lies in its ability to interact with the body's cardiovascular system in a targeted and controlled manner. The class of medications known as beta-adrenergic receptor blockers, or simply beta-blockers, includes this medication. Metoprolol tartrate lessens the effects of stress hormones by blocking particular heart receptors, which lowers blood pressure, slows the heart rate, and eventually lessens cardiac strain. Understanding how it works at a physiological level provides valuable insight into why it is such an essential tool in managing heart-related conditions.

The Role of Beta-Adrenergic Receptors
The body's response to stress is regulated by the autonomic nervous system, which includes the release of hormones like adrenaline (epinephrine) and noradrenaline (norepinephrine). These

hormones interact with beta-adrenergic receptors, which are proteins located on the surface of cells, especially in the heart, lungs, and blood vessels.

Beta receptors come in two primary varieties:
- **Beta-1 Receptors**: Primarily found in the heart, they increase heart rate, the force of contraction, and the release of renin (a hormone that raises blood pressure).
- **Beta-2 Receptors**: Found in the lungs and vascular smooth muscle, they control airway relaxation and dilation of blood vessels.

While these effects are beneficial during moments of acute stress (such as a fight-or-flight situation), prolonged activation of beta receptors can lead to harmful cardiovascular strain, particularly in people with conditions like hypertension, angina, or arrhythmias.

How Metoprolol Tartrate Works

As a selective beta-1 blocker, metoprolol tartrate mainly acts on the heart's beta-1 receptors. This is the step-by-step process:

1. Blocks Beta-1 Receptors in the Heart
- Adrenaline and noradrenaline cannot bind to beta-1 receptors when metoprolol is present. By doing so, it diminishes the effects of these stress hormones on the heart, leading to:
- The heart rate is slowed due to a negative chronotropic impact;
- This is caused by a decrease in the force of heart contractions (negative inotropic effect).
- Less oxygen demand by the heart, helping to alleviate chest pain (angina).

2. Reduces Blood Pressure

By lowering the heart rate and the force of contraction, Metoprolol decreases cardiac output the amount of blood the heart pumps with each beat. This reduction in cardiac output leads to a drop in blood pressure.

3. Suppresses Renin Release

Beta-1 receptors are also found in the kidneys, where they influence the release of renin, an enzyme that plays a key role in the body's regulation of blood pressure. By blocking these receptors, Metoprolol reduces renin release, which helps lower blood pressure further by inhibiting the renin-angiotensin-aldosterone system (RAAS).

4. Stabilizes Heart Rhythm

In conditions like arrhythmias, where the heart beats irregularly, Metoprolol helps restore a normal rhythm by reducing the excitability of heart tissue. It suppresses abnormal electrical signals that can cause irregular or rapid heartbeats, making it an effective treatment for conditions like atrial fibrillation or ventricular tachycardia.

Why Selectivity Matters

One important benefit of metoprolol is its specificity for beta-1 receptors. Unlike non-selective beta-blockers that also block beta-2 receptors, Metoprolol minimizes effects on the lungs and blood vessels. This selectivity makes it safer for patients with respiratory conditions such as asthma or chronic obstructive pulmonary disease (COPD), which can be exacerbated by beta-2 receptor blockade.

The Immediate-Release Advantage

As an immediate-release formulation, Metoprolol Tartrate acts quickly in the body, making it especially effective in acute situations like managing angina attacks or stabilizing heart rhythms during emergencies. However, this rapid action also means it must be taken more frequently (usually twice daily) to maintain its therapeutic effects.

Beyond the Heart

While the primary effects of Metoprolol Tartrate are on the heart, its action has systemic benefits:

- **Prevention of Migraines**: By modulating vascular tone and reducing the overactivity of certain brain signals, it can help prevent migraine attacks.
- **Management of Hyperthyroidism Symptoms:** By reducing the cardiovascular symptoms of hyperthyroidism, such as rapid heartbeat and tremors, Metoprolol Tartrate helps patients feel more stable.
- **Alleviation of Anxiety Symptoms**: In some cases, the calming effects of Metoprolol on heart rate and blood pressure can reduce the physical symptoms of anxiety, such as palpitations.

The Bigger Picture

Metoprolol Tartrate's mechanism of action exemplifies the elegance of modern pharmacology: a single molecule designed to target a specific receptor, yielding profound benefits for heart health and beyond. By slowing the heart, reducing its workload, and lowering blood pressure, Metoprolol Tartrate not only manages symptoms but also prevents long-term damage to the cardiovascular system.

Whether used to stabilize a life-threatening arrhythmia, protect the heart after a heart attack, or provide relief from chronic hypertension, the science behind Metoprolol Tartrate ensures it remains a critical player in the fight against cardiovascular disease. For patients, understanding how this medication works can provide peace of mind, helping them feel more confident in their treatment journey.

Pharmacokinetics of Metoprolol Tartrate

Pharmacokinetics explains how the body absorbs, distributes, metabolizes, and eliminates a substance. Understanding these processes for

Metoprolol Tartrate provides insights into how it works, how long it stays active in the system, and why it is administered in a specific manner. This knowledge not only helps healthcare providers optimize dosing but also allows patients to understand how the medication interacts with their bodies.

Absorption: How Metoprolol Tartrate Enters the Body

When taken orally, Metoprolol Tartrate is rapidly absorbed in the gastrointestinal (GI) tract. Its immediate-release formulation ensures that the drug reaches the bloodstream quickly, which is crucial for conditions requiring prompt action, such as angina or acute hypertension.

- **Bioavailability:**

The bioavailability of Metoprolol Tartrate how much of the drug reaches systemic circulation is approximately 50%. This is due to the first-pass metabolism in the liver, where a significant portion of the drug is metabolized before it enters the bloodstream.

- **Onset of Action:**

The effects of Metoprolol Tartrate are typically noticeable within 20–60 minutes after oral administration, making it effective for managing symptoms relatively quickly. Within 1.5 to 2 hours, peak plasma concentrations are reached.

Distribution: Where Metoprolol Travels in the Body

Once absorbed, Metoprolol Tartrate is distributed throughout the body, with a primary focus on tissues containing beta-1 adrenergic receptors, especially the heart.

- **Protein Binding:**

Metoprolol has a relatively low plasma protein binding rate (around 12%), meaning a significant portion of the drug remains free and active in the bloodstream. This low binding contributes to its effectiveness in reaching target tissues.

- **Volume of Distribution (Vd):**

The volume of distribution is approximately 3.2–5.6 L/kg, indicating that Metoprolol readily penetrates tissues, including the heart, liver, and kidneys.

- **Blood-Brain Barrier:**

Metoprolol is lipophilic, meaning it can cross the blood-brain barrier. This property is why it can sometimes affect the central nervous system (CNS), leading to side effects like fatigue or dizziness in some patients. However, this same characteristic also makes it effective for preventing migraines.

Metabolism: How the Body Processes Metoprolol

Metoprolol Tartrate is extensively metabolized in the liver by the cytochrome P450 enzyme system, specifically by the enzyme (CYP2D6).

- **Liver Metabolism:**

The liver converts Metoprolol into inactive metabolites, which means its therapeutic effects are primarily derived from the parent compound before metabolism occurs.

- **Genetic Variability**:

The activity of CYP2D6 can vary significantly between individuals due to genetic differences, classifying people as:
- large metabolizers (enzyme activity that is normal).
- Poor metabolizers (reduced enzyme activity), leading to higher drug levels and prolonged effects.
- Ultra-rapid metabolizers (increased enzyme activity), resulting in faster clearance and potentially reduced effectiveness.

These variations can influence how patients respond to Metoprolol, and in some cases, dosing adjustments may be necessary.

Excretion: How Metoprolol Leaves the Body
Metoprolol and its metabolites are primarily eliminated through the kidneys.

- **Renal Excretion:**

Approximately 95% of Metoprolol's metabolites are excreted in the urine. Since only around 5% of the drug is eliminated unaltered, the majority of it is digested before being eliminated.

- **Half-Life:**

The elimination half-life of Metoprolol Tartrate is relatively short, ranging from 3 to 7 hours in most individuals. This short half-life explains why it needs to be taken multiple times a day to maintain consistent therapeutic levels in the bloodstream.

- **Effect of Renal Impairment**:

In patients with impaired kidney function, the excretion of metabolites may be slower, but this has minimal impact on the drug's overall action since its therapeutic effects are mostly dictated by the parent substance.

Factors Affecting Pharmacokinetics

Several factors can influence how Metoprolol Tartrate is absorbed, metabolized, and excreted:

1. Age:

Older adults may experience slower metabolism and excretion, requiring adjustments in dosing to avoid excessive drug accumulation.

2. Liver Function:

Since Metoprolol is extensively metabolized in the liver, conditions like liver disease can significantly alter its pharmacokinetics, potentially leading to higher drug levels.

3. Drug Interactions:

Medications that inhibit or induce CYP2D6 can affect the metabolism of Metoprolol. For example:

- Inhibitors (e.g., fluoxetine, quinidine):Increase blood levels of Metoprolol, enhancing its effects and side effects.
- Inducers (e.g., rifampin): Reduce Metoprolol levels, potentially decreasing its effectiveness.

4. Food:

Taking Metoprolol Tartrate with food can slightly delay absorption but does not significantly impact its bioavailability or effectiveness.

Clinical Implications of Metoprolol's Pharmacokinetics

Comprehending the pharmacokinetics of metoprolol tartrate enables physicians to customize its administration for each patient. For instance:

- **Frequent Dosing:** The short half-life of Metoprolol Tartrate necessitates dosing 2–3 times daily to ensure steady therapeutic levels, particularly for conditions like angina or arrhythmias.
- **Personalized Therapy:** Genetic variability in CYP2D6 metabolism means some patients may require higher or lower doses for optimal effect.
- **Monitoring and Adjustments**: In patients with liver or kidney dysfunction, careful monitoring and dose adjustments are essential to avoid side effects.

A Seamless Balance Between Science and Therapy

Metoprolol Tartrate's pharmacokinetics reflect the sophistication of modern pharmacology. Its rapid absorption, effective tissue distribution, and predictable metabolism and excretion make it a reliable medication for managing cardiovascular conditions. This seamless interplay between its actions in the body and its therapeutic benefits underscores why Metoprolol Tartrate remains a cornerstone of heart health treatment today.

Dosage Forms of Metoprolol Tartrate

Metoprolol Tartrate, a cornerstone in the management of cardiovascular conditions, is available in various dosage forms to meet the needs of different medical scenarios. Whether used for routine blood pressure management, post-heart attack care, or acute interventions, these dosage options ensure flexibility and precision in treatment. Let's explore the available forms and how they cater to specific patient needs.

Oral Dosage Forms: The Most Commonly Used Option

Oral formulations of Metoprolol Tartrate are the primary choice for long-term management of conditions such as hypertension, angina, and arrhythmias.

1. Immediate-Release Tablets

Metoprolol Tartrate is primarily available as immediate-release tablets, designed for rapid absorption and action.

Available Strengths:
- 25 mg
- 50 mg
- 100 mg
- 200 mg

Key Features:
- The immediate-release formulation acts quickly, typically within 20–60 minutes after ingestion.
- Due to its short half-life (3–7 hours), it is generally prescribed for twice-daily dosing, ensuring stable blood levels.

Advantages:
- Suitable for conditions requiring prompt therapeutic effects, such as angina or arrhythmias.

- Healthcare professionals can customize treatment to meet the needs of each patient with flexible dosing.

2. Combination Tablets

In some cases, Metoprolol Tartrate is combined with other medications, such as diuretics, to enhance its effectiveness in treating hypertension. These combination tablets simplify treatment regimens by reducing the number of pills a patient needs to take daily.

Injectable Form: For Acute Medical Situations

Metoprolol Tartrate is also available as an injectable solution, used primarily in hospital or emergency settings.

Formulation:
- Injectable solution containing 1 mg/mL of Metoprolol Tartrate.

Administration:
- Delivered intravenously (IV), ensuring rapid action for acute situations where oral administration is not feasible or would take too long to act.
- Commonly administered under controlled conditions, with continuous monitoring of heart rate and blood pressure.

Indications:
- **Acute Myocardial Infarction (AMI)**: The injectable form is used to stabilize patients experiencing a heart attack by quickly reducing heart rate and cardiac workload.
- **Severe Arrhythmias**: Provides immediate control of life-threatening irregular heart rhythms.

Advantages:
- Rapid onset of action makes it ideal for emergency use.

- Accurate titration to produce the intended therapeutic effect is ensured by precise dosage.

Special Dosage Forms in Development

While the primary forms of Metoprolol Tartrate are tablets and injectables, researchers and pharmaceutical companies continue to explore new formulations. These innovations aim to improve patient compliance, enhance convenience, and expand its therapeutic applications.

Orally Disintegrating Tablets (ODTs):

These dissolve in the mouth without water, offering convenience for patients who have difficulty swallowing traditional tablets.

Transdermal Patches:

Although not yet widely available, transdermal patches delivering Metoprolol could provide a once-daily option, improving adherence for patients with busy lifestyles or complex medication regimens.

Choosing the Right Dosage Form

The choice of dosage form depends on several factors, including:

1. Condition Being Treated:
- Immediate-release tablets are suitable for chronic management.
- Injectable solutions are reserved for emergencies.

2. Patient Preference and Compliance:
- Some patients may prefer smaller doses taken multiple times a day, while others might benefit from combination tablets to reduce pill burden.

3. Medical Setting:
- In hospitals, the injectable form is preferred for immediate therapeutic effects.

Personalized Dosing for Optimal Outcomes

Metoprolol Tartrate's versatility in dosage forms allows healthcare providers to customize treatment plans to individual needs. This flexibility ensures that each patient receives the most effective and convenient therapy possible.

For example:
- A patient recovering from a heart attack might start with the injectable form in the hospital, followed by oral tablets upon discharge.
- Someone managing chronic hypertension might benefit from twice-daily immediate-release tablets or a combination pill.

CHAPTER THREE

Primary Indications of Metoprolol Tartrate

Metoprolol Tartrate is a highly effective medication that plays a critical role in managing several cardiovascular conditions. By working on the heart and blood vessels, it helps reduce the workload on the heart, control blood pressure, and stabilize heart rhythms. Below, we will dive deeper into the primary conditions for which Metoprolol Tartrate is commonly prescribed: "Hypertension", "Angina Pectoris", "Post-Myocardial Infarction Care", and "Arrhythmias".

1. Hypertension (High Blood Pressure)

A common yet dangerous disorder known as hypertension occurs when the artery's blood pressure is continuously too high.

It can result in serious side effects like kidney failure, heart disease, and stroke if left untreated.

Metoprolol Tartrate is commonly used in the management of hypertension due to its ability to reduce heart rate and cardiac output.

How Metoprolol Helps in Hypertension:
- **Reduces Heart Rate**: By blocking beta-1 receptors in the heart, Metoprolol decreases the heart rate (negative chronotropic effect), reducing the amount of work the heart has to do to pump blood.
- **Lowers Blood Pressure**: By reducing the force of heart contractions (negative inotropic effect), Metoprolol decreases cardiac output, leading to a decrease in blood pressure.
- **Symptom Relief:** High blood pressure often doesn't cause symptoms, but Metoprolol helps patients feel more comfortable by stabilizing heart function.

Why It's Effective:

Metoprolol is often prescribed for patients with primary (essential) hypertension as well as secondary hypertension, where high blood pressure is caused by other underlying conditions like kidney disease. By lowering both systolic and diastolic blood pressure, Metoprolol reduces the risk of long-term complications like stroke, heart attack, and organ damage.

2. Angina Pectoris (Chest Pain)

When the heart muscle does not receive enough oxygen-rich blood, it can cause angina pectoris, which is a pain or discomfort in the chest. It often results from narrowed coronary arteries due to atherosclerosis. While angina itself is not a heart attack, it signals that the heart is under stress. Metoprolol Tartrate is an essential tool in managing this condition by reducing the heart's oxygen demand.

How Metoprolol Helps in Angina:
- **Decreases Heart Rate and Oxygen Demand:** Metoprolol lowers the heart rate and reduces the strength of heart contractions, thus requiring less oxygen to perform its functions.
- **Improves Exercise Tolerance**: By controlling heart rate and reducing ischemic episodes (lack of oxygen), Metoprolol helps patients engage in physical activities without triggering chest pain.
- Reduces Frequency of Angina Attacks: By stabilizing the heart's workload, Metoprolol can significantly reduce the frequency and severity of angina episodes, improving quality of life.

Why It's Effective:
Metoprolol is considered a cornerstone in the treatment of chronic stable angina. It is often prescribed in combination with other medications like nitrates or calcium channel blockers to

maximize symptom relief. This combination helps open up the coronary arteries, improving blood flow and oxygen delivery to the heart, while Metoprolol manages the heart's response to physical stress.

3. Post-Myocardial Infarction Care (Heart Attack Recovery)

A myocardial infarction (MI), another name for a heart attack, occurs when a blood clot blocks blood flow to the heart muscle, causing damage to the tissue. After a heart attack, it's critical to reduce the heart's workload and prevent further complications, including another heart attack. Metoprolol Tartrate is widely used in post-MI care to help stabilize the heart and improve long-term recovery.

How Metoprolol Helps After a Heart Attack:
- **Prevents Further Damage**: By reducing heart rate and contractility, Metoprolol minimizes the heart's oxygen demand,

allowing the healing heart muscle to recover more effectively.

- **Reduces Risk of Arrhythmias**: Following a heart attack, patients are at increased risk for dangerous arrhythmias. Metoprolol helps stabilize the heart rhythm, reducing the risk of sudden cardiac death.
- **Improves Survival Rates**: Clinical studies have shown that patients who take Metoprolol following a heart attack have improved survival rates and fewer complications. It helps prevent further myocardial damage and promotes long-term heart health.

Why It's Effective:
Metoprolol is part of evidence-based guidelines for the treatment of acute myocardial infarction and its aftermath. By decreasing the workload on the heart, Metoprolol allows the heart muscle time to heal while minimizing the chances of complications like heart failure or recurrent heart attacks.

4. Arrhythmias (Irregular Heart Rhythms)

Arrhythmias refer to abnormal heart rhythms, which can either be too fast, too slow, or erratic. Ventricular tachycardia, atrial fibrillation, and atrial flutter are common forms. These conditions can be life-threatening if not managed properly. Metoprolol Tartrate is frequently used to treat arrhythmias due to its ability to regulate heart rate and rhythm.

How Metoprolol Helps in Arrhythmias:
- **Slows Down the Heart Rate**: Metoprolol slows the heart rate by blocking beta-1 receptors, making it effective in treating tachycardia (rapid heart rate) and other arrhythmias.
- **Restores Normal Heart Rhythm**: In conditions like atrial fibrillation, Metoprolol helps restore a more regular rhythm by controlling the conduction of electrical signals through the heart.

- **Reduces Risk of Complications**: By controlling arrhythmias, Metoprolol reduces the risk of stroke, heart failure, and sudden cardiac arrest, all of which can occur as a result of untreated or poorly controlled arrhythmias.

Why It's Effective:
For patients with chronic arrhythmias like atrial fibrillation, Metoprolol is often used long-term to maintain a stable heart rhythm. For those with acute arrhythmic episodes, it is often used in the short term, particularly in a hospital setting, to restore normal rhythm and prevent complications.

Metoprolol tartrate is a multipurpose and necessary drug for treating a variety of heart diseases. The most common reasons it is prescribed are:

- Hypertension: Reduces blood pressure and prevents long-term complications like stroke and heart failure.

- Angina Pectoris: Relieves chest pain and improves exercise tolerance by reducing the heart's oxygen demand.
- Post-Myocardial Infarction Care: Improves survival rates and heart recovery after a heart attack.
- Arrhythmias: Stabilizes the heart rhythm, reducing the risk of life-threatening arrhythmic events.

For each of these conditions, Metoprolol Tartrate is not only effective in alleviating symptoms but also plays a crucial role in preventing further complications and improving long-term heart health. It remains one of the most trusted medications in modern cardiovascular therapy.

Off-Label Uses of Metoprolol Tartrate

While Metoprolol Tartrate is primarily prescribed for cardiovascular conditions, such as hypertension, angina, and arrhythmias, it has also found success in treating a variety of other health issues, even though these uses are not officially approved by regulatory bodies like the U.S. FDA. These **off-label uses** allow patients to benefit from Metoprolol in treating conditions like migraine prevention and **anxiety-related disorders**, expanding the versatility of this medication beyond its typical applications.

1. Migraine Prevention

Migraine headaches are intense, recurring headaches often accompanied by nausea, vomiting, and sensitivity to light and sound. While the exact cause of migraines is not fully understood, it is believed that changes in the brain's blood vessels and neurotransmitter activity contribute to their onset. Although Metoprolol is not FDA-approved specifically for the prevention of migraines, it has been shown to be an effective treatment for reducing the frequency and severity of these episodes.

How Metoprolol Helps Prevent Migraines:
- **Vascular Stabilization**:

It is believed that the dilatation and constriction of blood vessels in the brain are linked to migraines. Metoprolol, as a beta-blocker, can stabilize the blood vessels, preventing the changes in vascular tone that contribute to migraine onset.

- **Decrease in sympathetic nervous system activity:**

Metoprolol works by blocking beta-adrenergic receptors, particularly the beta-1 receptors in the heart and brain. By inhibiting the overactivity of the sympathetic nervous system (which can trigger migraine episodes), it helps reduce the frequency of attacks.

- **CNS Effects**:

Metoprolol's ability to cross the blood-brain barrier means it can directly influence the central nervous system. This action may help reduce the brain's heightened sensitivity to stimuli, which is a common feature of migraines.

Why It's Effective:

Studies have shown that beta-blockers like Metoprolol can be effective in reducing the frequency of migraines by about 30-50%. They are generally considered a first-line treatment for migraine prophylaxis, particularly for individuals who experience frequent or chronic migraines.

Metoprolol's low incidence of side effects compared to other migraine medications (like triptans or NSAIDs) makes it a favorable option for many patients looking for long-term prevention strategies.

Dosage for Migraine Prevention:

The typical dosage for migraine prevention is lower than the dose used for hypertension or heart-related conditions, often starting at **50 mg** per day and adjusted based on individual needs. Patients may need to take it daily for several weeks before noticing a reduction in migraine frequency.

2. Anxiety-Related Conditions

Metoprolol is sometimes prescribed for anxiety-related conditions, particularly for situational anxiety and performance anxiety. These conditions involve physiological symptoms, such as rapid heart rate, trembling, sweating, and palpitations, which are triggered by stress or anxiety-inducing situations. While Metoprolol is not FDA-approved for anxiety disorders, its ability to control the physical symptoms associated with anxiety makes it a useful off-label option.

How Metoprolol Helps in Anxiety:
- **Control of Physical Symptoms:**

Anxiety often triggers a "fight or flight" response in the body, which includes an increase in heart rate and blood pressure. Metoprolol, as a beta-blocker, works by blocking the beta-1 receptors in the heart, leading to a reduction in heart rate and blood pressure. This aids in reducing the bodily manifestations of anxiety, like shaking or a racing heart.

- **Improved Psychological Calm:**

By controlling the physiological symptoms that can amplify feelings of anxiety, Metoprolol helps patients feel more at ease in stressful situations. It is especially useful in performance anxiety, where individuals experience overwhelming nervousness or fear of public speaking or performing.

- **No Sedation or Cognitive Impact**

Unlike benzodiazepines (another class of medications commonly prescribed for anxiety), Metoprolol does not cause sedation or impair cognitive function. This makes it particularly appealing for patients who need to stay alert and focused while managing anxiety symptoms.

Why It's Effective:

For patients with **situational anxiety** (e.g., anxiety related to public speaking, presentations, or performances), Metoprolol provides rapid relief of physical symptoms without causing drowsiness or cognitive impairment. It is often used on an as-needed basis before stressful events, helping patients feel more in control.

Dosage for Anxiety-Related Conditions:

For situational anxiety or performance anxiety, Metoprolol is typically taken at a lower dose of **25 mg to 50 mg** about an hour before the stressful event. For long-term management of anxiety disorders, other medications or therapies may be considered in conjunction with or instead of Metoprolol.

Why These Off-Label Uses Matter

Both migraine prevention and anxiety-related conditions can significantly affect a person's quality of life, and traditional treatments may not always work for every patient. Off-label uses of Metoprolol Tartrate offer an alternative option for individuals seeking relief from these conditions.

- Non-Sedating: Unlike many anxiety medications, Metoprolol doesn't cause drowsiness or mental fog, making it a better

choice for people who need to remain active and productive.
- Minimal Side Effects: Metoprolol is generally well-tolerated with a relatively low incidence of side effects, especially when compared to other medications that may have more pronounced adverse effects.
- Dual Benefits: The fact that Metoprolol can be used to manage both cardiovascular conditions and conditions like migraines or anxiety demonstrates its versatility, allowing patients with multiple issues to benefit from one medication.

CHAPTER FOUR:
Administration and Dosage

Guidelines for Use of Metoprolol Tartrate

When it comes to Metoprolol Tartrate, proper dosing and frequency are essential to ensure that the medication is effective, while minimizing the risk of side effects. This section provides a comprehensive guide on how Metoprolol should be used, including key recommendations for its dosing, frequency, and considerations for individual patients.

1. Dosing for Different Conditions

The dose of Metoprolol Tartrate varies depending on the condition being treated, the patient's response to the medication, and other individual factors like age and overall health. The goal is to use the **lowest effective dose** that provides the desired therapeutic effects while minimizing potential side effects

Hypertension (High Blood Pressure)

For hypertension, Metoprolol is typically started at a low dose to assess tolerance and effectiveness, and then adjusted based on the patient's response.

Initial Dose:
- The usual starting dose for adults is 50 mg once daily.
- Some patients may start at a lower dose of 25 mg depending on their condition and other health factors, such as kidney function.

Maintenance Dose:
- The maintenance dosage varies based on the patient's blood pressure response, ranging from 50 mg to 200 mg daily.
- Doses can be split into two daily doses if necessary, particularly for patients who

require higher amounts (e.g., 100 mg taken as 50 mg twice a day).

Max Dose:
For some patients, particularly those who do not respond adequately to lower doses, the dose may be increased gradually. The maximum recommended dose for hypertension is 400 mg/day, although this is uncommon and typically reserved for those with significant blood pressure issues.

Angina Pectoris (Chest Pain)
For angina, Metoprolol helps reduce heart rate and oxygen demand, preventing chest pain by reducing the strain on the heart.

Initial Dose:
- The typical starting dose for angina is 50 mg once daily.

Maintenance Dose:
- Depending on the severity of symptoms, the dose may be increased to 100 mg to 200 mg

per day, usually split into two doses (e.g., 100 mg twice daily).

Max Dose:
- The maximum dose for managing angina is typically around 400 mg/day, but this would be rare and should be carefully monitored by a healthcare provider.

Post-Myocardial Infarction (Post-Heart Attack Care)

Following a heart attack, Metoprolol is used to prevent further complications, such as arrhythmias or additional heart damage.

Initial Dose:
- Following a heart attack, the usual starting dose is 25 mg to 50 mg twice daily.

Maintenance Dose:
- Gradual adjustments are made to reach a maintenance dose of 100 mg to 200 mg per day, divided into two doses.

Max Dose:
- The maximum dose for post-heart attack care typically does not exceed 200 mg/day, divided into two doses.

Arrhythmias (Irregular Heart Rhythms)
For arrhythmias, Metoprolol is used to control heart rate and rhythm, reducing the occurrence of dangerous irregularities.

Initial Dose:
- For arrhythmias, the starting dose is often 25 mg to 50 mg twice a day.

Maintenance Dose:
- Doses are typically adjusted depending on the patient's heart rate and the severity of the arrhythmia. Two daily doses of 50 mg to 200 mg are typical maintenance dosages.

Max Dose:
- The maximum recommended dose for arrhythmias is 400 mg/day, but this dose is

usually only necessary in severe cases or when managing arrhythmias that are difficult to control.

2. Considerations for Special Populations

Certain patient groups may require adjustments to the standard dosing of Metoprolol Tartrate, including the elderly, those with renal or hepatic impairment, and those with other underlying conditions. It's crucial for healthcare providers to monitor these patients carefully to ensure safe and effective use.

Elderly Patients

Metoprolol may have more of an impact on older folks, especially when it comes to blood pressure and heart rate. As a result, the initial dose should be lower, often starting at 25 mg per day. The dose can then be gradually increased based on tolerance and response.

Renal Impairment

Patients with renal impairment (kidney disease) may require careful monitoring and dose adjustments, as Metoprolol is excreted through the kidneys. The dose should be started at the lower end of the range, such as 25 mg, and adjusted as necessary based on kidney function. In cases of severe renal impairment, the healthcare provider may opt for a more conservative dosing approach.

Hepatic Impairment
Metoprolol is metabolized in the liver, so patients with liver dysfunction may need lower starting doses. The initial dose might be 25 mg per day, with gradual adjustments based on individual tolerance and response

3. Dosing for Off-Label Uses
In some cases, Metoprolol may be prescribed off-label for conditions like migraine prevention or anxiety-related symptoms, which require different dosing strategies than those used for heart conditions.

Migraine Prevention:
- The typical starting dose for migraine prevention is 50 mg once daily, with adjustments based on effectiveness and tolerability. Some patients may require up to 100 mg per day.

Anxiety Management:
- For performance anxiety or situational anxiety, Metoprolol is typically taken 30 to 60 minutes before the anxiety-inducing event. The usual dose ranges from 25 mg to 50 mg.

4. Key Points for Proper Use
- **Consistency in Dosing:**

Metoprolol Tartrate should be taken at the same time each day, with or without food, to maintain consistent blood levels. This helps ensure that the medication remains effective and the patient avoids missing doses.

- **Swallowing the Tablets:**

Metoprolol pills should be taken whole by patients with a glass of water. Do not chew or crush the tablets, as this can alter the way the medication is absorbed by the body.

- **Missed Dose:**

If a dose is missed, the patient should take it as soon as they remember, unless it's almost time for the next dose. lightheadedness or dizziness, especially when standing up fast.

- **Gradual Dose Adjustments**:

Doses should be increased gradually to avoid potential side effects like low blood pressure or an excessively slow heart rate. Always follow the healthcare provider's recommendations and avoid self-adjusting the dose.

Monitoring: Regular monitoring of heart rate, blood pressure, and ECG (electrocardiogram) is important during Metoprolol therapy, especially during dose adjustments or if the patient experiences side effects. It helps ensure that the drug is working as intended and not causing adverse effects.

5. Side Effects to Watch For

Although Metoprolol is generally well tolerated, patients should be aware of potential side effects, particularly if the dose is too high. These may include:

- lightheadedness or dizziness, especially when standing up fast.
- Fatigue or weakness.
- Slow heart rate (bradycardia), which may need to be managed by adjusting the dose.
- Shortness of breath or swelling, which may indicate heart failure in some patients.

If any of these occur, patients should contact their healthcare provider for advice.

Special Populations and Metoprolol Tartrate

While Metoprolol Tartrate is a widely used medication with proven efficacy in treating conditions like hypertension, angina, and arrhythmias, special populations such as the elderly, children, and individuals with kidney or liver impairments require particular attention when it comes to dosing and management. This section will provide a detailed guide on how Metoprolol Tartrate should be used in these populations to ensure safety and effectiveness.

1. The Elderly: Special Considerations for Older Adults

Older adults often have different physiological responses to medications compared to younger populations. Metoprolol Tartrate is no exception, and dosing adjustments are necessary to ensure both efficacy and safety in elderly patients.

Challenges in the Elderly:

- **Decreased organ function**: As people age, their kidney and liver function may decline, which can affect how the body processes medications. This may result in a slower rate of drug clearance and a higher chance of adverse consequences.
- **Polypharmacy**: Elderly individuals often take multiple medications for various chronic conditions, which can lead to drug interactions and an increased risk of adverse effects.
- **Increased sensitivity:** Older adults may be more sensitive to beta-blockers, particularly in terms of blood pressure and heart rate regulation.

Dosing Recommendations:
- **Starting Dose**:

For elderly patients, the starting dose is typically lower than the standard adult dose. A common starting dose is 25 mg to 50 mg once daily.

- **Gradual Adjustments**:

The dose should be increased gradually based on the patient's response and tolerance. Monitoring of heart rate, blood pressure, and renal function is essential when adjusting the dose.

- **Maximum Dose**:

The maximum dose in elderly patients is generally 200 mg per day, However, in order to lessen the danger of bradycardia (slow heart rate) and hypotension (low blood pressure), doses are usually kept on the lower end of the spectrum.

Monitoring and Caution:
- Close monitoring for signs of orthostatic hypotension (a sudden drop in blood pressure when standing up) is important, as older adults are more prone to dizziness and falls.
- Monitor renal and hepatic function regularly, as any changes could require further dose adjustments.

2. Children: Use in Pediatric Populations

Metoprolol Tartrate is generally not the first-line treatment for children, but it may be prescribed for certain pediatric conditions, particularly those involving congenital heart defects, arrhythmias, or hypertrophic cardiomyopathy.

Challenges in Children:
- **Dosage variations**: Children's metabolic rates differ significantly from adults, and this can affect how drugs are absorbed, distributed, and eliminated. For children, the appropriate dose needs to be carefully determined by a pediatrician.
- **Limited data**: The safety and effectiveness of Metoprolol in pediatric populations have not been as extensively studied as in adults, so the prescribing physician must rely on clinical judgment and experience.

Dosing Recommendations for Children:

Starting Dose:

For pediatric patients, the starting dose of Metoprolol Tartrate is usually 0.5 mg to 1 mg per kg of body weight, administered once or twice daily.

Maintenance Dose:

The dose may be gradually increased to a maintenance dose of 1 mg to 2 mg per kg of body weight per day, divided into two doses, depending on the child's age, weight, and condition being treated.

Maximum Dose:

The maximum daily dose for children typically does not exceed 4 mg per kg of body weight, but again, this depends on the child's specific health circumstances and the prescribing healthcare provider's recommendations.

Monitoring and Caution:
- Because children may be more sensitive to beta-blockers, it is important to monitor for

side effects such as slow heart rate (bradycardia), fatigue, or hypotension.
- Regular electrocardiograms (ECGs) should be performed to monitor the heart's rhythm, especially in children with arrhythmias or heart conditions.

3. Kidney Impairment: Adjustments for Renal Dysfunction

Metoprolol Tartrate is partially excreted through the kidneys, so patients with impaired renal function may require dosage adjustments to avoid the buildup of the medication in the body. Kidney dysfunction can lead to the slower elimination of Metoprolol, increasing the risk of adverse effects.

Challenges in Renal Impairment:
- **Slower clearance**: In individuals with kidney impairment, Metoprolol may not be eliminated as quickly from the body, leading to an increased concentration of the drug in the bloodstream.

- Risk of toxicity: Without proper dosing adjustments, kidney impairment can increase the likelihood of experiencing side effects such as bradycardia, hypotension, or fatigue.

Dosing Recommendations:

Mild to Moderate Renal Impairment:

In patients with mild to moderate kidney impairment (e.g., creatinine clearance of 30–60 mL/min), the starting dose should generally be lower than the typical dose, often starting at 25 mg once daily. This can be gradually increased depending on the patient's tolerance and kidney function.

Severe Renal Impairment:

In cases of severe renal impairment (e.g., creatinine clearance less than 30 mL/min), the use of Metoprolol should be closely monitored. The dose is usually kept at the lower end of the dosing range and might be reduced further, with doses of 25 mg per day or even less, depending on the patient's clinical condition.

Monitoring and Caution:
- Kidney function should be regularly monitored, especially in patients with advanced renal disease. Serum creatinine and creatinine clearance levels are important indicators of how the kidneys are processing the medication.
- Be vigilant for signs of fluid retention or worsening kidney function, which could necessitate dose adjustments or even discontinuation of the medication.

4. Liver Impairment: Adjustments for Hepatic Dysfunction

Metoprolol is metabolized in the liver, so patients with liver impairments may experience slower clearance and higher concentrations of the drug in their system. A lower dosage and closer observation may be necessary for those who have liver problems.

Challenges in Liver Impairment:
- **Altered metabolism**: Liver dysfunction can affect the enzymes that metabolize Metoprolol, leading to higher drug levels in the bloodstream and an increased risk of adverse effects.
- Potential for drug interactions: Individuals with liver disease are often on multiple medications, and the liver's reduced capacity for drug metabolism may increase the risk of dangerous interactions.

Dosing Recommendations

Mild to Moderate Hepatic Impairment:

For patients with mild to moderate liver disease, Metoprolol should typically be started at a lower dose, such as 25 mg per day. The dose can be gradually increased depending on how the patient responds to the medication.

Severe Hepatic Impairment:

For patients with severe liver impairment, Metoprolol should be used cautiously, often starting at 25 mg or lower. In these cases, dose adjustments should be made with extra care, and patients should be closely monitored for side effects, such as bradycardia or hypotension.

Monitoring and Caution:
- Liver function should be regularly monitored, particularly in those with cirrhosis or active liver disease. Liver enzyme levels (such as ALT and AST) can provide insights into the liver's ability to metabolize the medication.

- Special attention should be paid to drug interactions, especially with other medications metabolized in the liver, to avoid the potential for drug toxicity.

Tailoring Metoprolol Treatment to Special Populations

While Metoprolol Tartrate is a highly effective medication for managing cardiovascular conditions, its use must be carefully tailored for special populations, including the elderly, children, and those with renal or liver impairment. By adjusting the dosage based on individual health factors and closely monitoring for side effects, healthcare providers can ensure that Metoprolol remains a safe and effective treatment for patients with unique needs. Always consult with a healthcare professional before starting or adjusting Metoprolol therapy to ensure the best possible outcome.

Drug Interactions with Metoprolol Tartrate

When taking any medication, it's crucial to be aware of potential **drug interactions**, as these can affect how well the medication works or increase the risk of side effects. Metoprolol Tartrate, like many medications, can interact with a variety of substances, including other medications, supplements, and even food. This section will provide a detailed overview of the key drug interactions with Metoprolol Tartrate, helping you understand how these interactions could impact your treatment.

1. Drugs That Increase the Effects of Metoprolol Tartrate

Some medications can enhance the effects of Metoprolol, increasing the risk of adverse reactions such as low heart rate (bradycardia), low blood pressure (hypotension), and fatigue. These drugs should be used cautiously in combination with

Metoprolol, and often require careful monitoring by healthcare professionals.

Calcium Channel Blockers (e.g., Verapamil, Diltiazem)

- Effect: Both Metoprolol and calcium channel blockers like verapamil and diltiazem can lower heart rate and blood pressure. When combined, they can lead to excessive bradycardia (slow heart rate) or hypotension (low blood pressure).
- Management: Co-administration should be done cautiously, and the patient's heart rate and blood pressure should be closely monitored. Sometimes, the doses of one or both medications may need to be adjusted.

Antiarrhythmic Drugs (e.g., Amiodarone, Sotalol)

- Effect: Antiarrhythmics such as amiodarone and sotalol work by stabilizing heart rhythms, but they also have a slowing effect

on the heart rate. When taken with Metoprolol, there is a risk of **severe bradycardia or other rhythm disturbances.
- Management: If these drugs are prescribed alongside Metoprolol, the healthcare provider may opt for a lower dose of either medication and will carefully monitor the patient's heart rhythm, blood pressure, and other vital signs.

Alpha-Blockers (e.g., Prazosin, Doxazosin)
- Effect: Alpha-blockers, which are used to treat hypertension, can lower blood pressure by dilating blood vessels. When combined with Metoprolol, the risk of severe hypotension increases, particularly when standing up (orthostatic hypotension).
- Management: Blood pressure should be monitored closely, especially during the initial stages of therapy or dose adjustments. If necessary, the dose of either Metoprolol or the alpha-blocker may be reduced.

Antihypertensive Medications (e.g., Clonidine, ACE Inhibitors, Diuretics)
- Effect: Other antihypertensive agents, such as clonidine (a centrally acting antihypertensive) and ACE inhibitors, can potentiate the blood-pressure-lowering effects of Metoprolol.
- Management: Combining these medications with Metoprolol requires careful titration to avoid excessively low blood pressure. Regular monitoring of blood pressure is essential.

Insulin and Oral Hypoglycemic Agents
- Effect: Metoprolol may mask symptoms of hypoglycemia(low blood sugar) such as tremors, palpitations, and anxiety, making it harder for people with diabetes to recognize when their blood sugar is too low.
- Management: Close monitoring of blood glucose levels is recommended when

Metoprolol is used in diabetic patients. The patient may need adjustments to their diabetes treatment regimen.

2. Drugs That Decrease the Effectiveness of Metoprolol Tartrate

Some medications can reduce the effectiveness of Metoprolol, potentially compromising its ability to manage conditions like hypertension or arrhythmias.

Nonsteroidal Anti-Inflammatory Drugs (NSAIDs, e.g., Ibuprofen, Naproxen)

- Effect: NSAIDs, such as ibuprofen and naproxen, can counteract the blood pressure-lowering effects of Metoprolol by causing fluid retention and constricting blood vessels.
- Management: While occasional use of NSAIDs may not significantly interfere with Metoprolol, chronic use should be avoided,

especially in patients being treated for high blood pressure. If NSAIDs are needed, the patient should be closely monitored for any changes in blood pressure.

Rifampin (Antibiotic)
- Effect: Rifampin is an antibiotic that can accelerate the metabolism of Metoprolol in the liver, leading to a reduced plasma concentration and thus a decrease in its effectiveness.
- Management: If rifampin is prescribed, higher doses of Metoprolol may be required, but this should only be done under the guidance of a healthcare provider. It is recommended to regularly check heart rate and blood pressure.

Barbiturates (e.g., Phenobarbital)
- Effect: Barbiturates like phenobarbital can induce liver enzymes, speeding up the

metabolism of Metoprolol and potentially reducing its effectiveness.
- Management: Dosage adjustments may be needed if Metoprolol is prescribed alongside barbiturates. The healthcare provider will monitor the patient's response to ensure therapeutic levels are maintained.

3. Drugs That Increase the Risk of Metoprolol Tartrate Side Effects

Certain medications can increase the risk of side effects when taken with Metoprolol, including dizziness, fatigue, and heart-related issues. These drugs require careful consideration when prescribed together.

Antidepressants (e.g., Fluoxetine, Paroxetine)

- Effect: Selective serotonin reuptake inhibitors (SSRIs) such as fluoxetine and paroxetine can increase the levels of Metoprolol in the blood, possibly leading to

enhanced side effects like bradycardia and hypotension
- Management: If an SSRI is prescribed alongside Metoprolol, the patient should be closely monitored for signs of excessive slowing of the heart rate or a significant drop in blood pressure. The healthcare provider may consider dose adjustments.

Digoxin (for Heart Failure or Arrhythmias)
- Effect: Digoxin is used to treat heart failure and arrhythmias, and when combined with Metoprolol, it can increase the risk of heart block or bradycardia (slow heart rate). The combination may make the heart's electrical conduction system more susceptible to disturbances.
- Management: This combination should only be used under strict medical supervision, with regular monitoring of electrocardiograms (ECGs) and heart rate. It

could be necessary to change the dosage of one or both drugs.

Alcohol
- Effect: Alcohol can potentiate the blood-pressure-lowering effects of Metoprolol, leading to dizziness, lightheadedness, or fainting. Alcohol can also impair the liver's ability to metabolize medications, potentially leading to higher drug levels in the bloodstream.
- Management: Patients should be advised to limit alcohol consumption while taking Metoprolol, and they should avoid drinking large amounts, particularly when starting or adjusting the medication.

Challenges in Liver Impairment:
- Altered metabolism: Liver dysfunction can affect the enzymes that metabolize Metoprolol, leading to higher drug levels in

the bloodstream and an increased risk of adverse effects.
- Potential for drug interactions Individuals with liver disease are often on multiple medications, and the liver's reduced capacity for drug metabolism may increase the risk of dangerous interactions.

Dosing Recommendations

Mild to Moderate Hepatic Impairment:

For patients with mild to moderate liver disease, Metoprolol should typically be started at a lower dose, such as 25 mg per day. The dose can be gradually increased depending on how the patient responds to the medication.

Severe Hepatic Impairment:

For patients with severe liver impairment, Metoprolol should be used cautiously, often starting at 25 mg or lower. In these cases, dose adjustments should be made with extra care, and patients should be closely monitored for side effects, such as bradycardia or hypotension.

Monitoring and Caution:
- Liver function should be regularly monitored, particularly in those with cirrhosis or active liver disease. Liver enzyme levels (such as ALT and AST) can provide insights into the liver's ability to metabolize the medication.
- Special attention should be paid to drug interactions, especially with other medications metabolized in the liver, to avoid the potential for drug toxicity.

Tailoring Metoprolol Treatment to Special Populations

While Metoprolol Tartrate is a highly effective medication for managing cardiovascular conditions, its use must be carefully tailored for special populations, including the elderly, children, and those with renal or liver impairment. By adjusting the dosage based on individual health factors and closely monitoring for side effects, healthcare providers can ensure that Metoprolol remains a safe and effective treatment for patients with unique needs. Always consult with a healthcare professional before starting or adjusting Metoprolol therapy to ensure the best possible outcome.

CHAPTER FIVE: Side Effects and Risks

Common Side Effects of Metoprolol Tartrate

Metoprolol tartrate, a widely prescribed beta-blocker, effectively manages conditions like hypertension, angina, and certain cardiac arrhythmias. It may, however, have adverse effects, just like any medication. Among the most commonly reported are fatigue, dizziness, and bradycardia. Below is an expanded exploration of these effects to provide readers with a deeper understanding.

1. Fatigue

One of the most frequently reported side effects of metoprolol tartrate is a sensation of fatigue or tiredness.

- **Why it happens**: The drug slows the heart rate and reduces the workload on the heart,

which is beneficial for conditions like hypertension or heart failure. However, this can sometimes lead to reduced oxygen and nutrient supply to muscles, causing a sense of sluggishness or lack of energy.
- **Patient experience**: Many patients describe this fatigue as a pervasive tiredness, even after a full night's sleep. It can affect daily activities, making tasks like climbing stairs or prolonged standing feel more strenuous.

Management tips
- Adjusting the timing of the medication (e.g., taking it at night) can sometimes help.
- Staying hydrated and engaging in light physical activities, such as walking, may counteract mild fatigue.
- If fatigue is severe or persistent, consult a healthcare provider, as dose adjustments or alternative medications might be necessary.

2. Dizziness

Dizziness, especially when standing up too quickly, is another common side effect. This is often due to the drug's impact on blood pressure.

- **Why it happens**: Metoprolol lowers blood pressure, which can sometimes lead to orthostatic hypotension a sudden drop in blood pressure upon standing. This results in dizziness or lightheadedness.
- **Patient experience**: Some individuals report feeling unsteady, while others describe brief moments of vertigo. In rare cases, dizziness can lead to fainting.

Management tips:

- Rising slowly from a sitting or lying position can minimize dizziness.
- Drinking plenty of fluids and avoiding dehydration is crucial.
- Avoiding alcohol and other substances that lower blood pressure can also reduce symptoms.

3. Bradycardia (Slow Heart Rate)

Metoprolol's intended effect is to slow down the heart rate, but in some cases, it can reduce the rate excessively, leading to bradycardia.

- **Why it happens**: The medication blocks beta-adrenergic receptors, decreasing the heart's response to stress hormones like adrenaline. While this is beneficial in treating arrhythmias and angina, it may slow the heart rate below normal levels (typically <60 beats per minute).
- **Patient experience**: Bradycardia might be asymptomatic in some, but others may feel faint, experience shortness of breath, or have difficulty exercising.

Management tips:
- Regularly monitoring your heart rate, especially during the initial phase of treatment, can help detect bradycardia early.
- Consult your doctor if you experience symptoms like fainting or extreme fatigue, as the dosage may need adjustment.

When to Seek Medical Attention

While these side effects are generally mild and manageable, some cases may require immediate medical attention. Seek help if you experience:

- Severe dizziness or fainting.
- Persistent fatigue that affects your quality of life.
- Extremely slow heart rate accompanied by chest pain or difficulty breathing.

Severe Risks of Metoprolol Tartrate

While metoprolol tartrate is an effective and commonly used medication for managing cardiovascular conditions, it can, in rare instances, lead to severe risks. Two significant risks are bronchospasms and worsening heart failure. Understanding these complications is crucial for patients and healthcare providers to ensure safe and effective use.

1. Bronchospasms

Bronchospasms are a severe tightening of the muscles around the airways, leading to breathing difficulties.

- **Why it happens:**

Metoprolol is a selective beta-1 adrenergic receptor blocker, primarily affecting the heart. However, at higher doses, it can lose selectivity and block beta-2 adrenergic receptors, which are present in the lungs. This unintended effect can cause airway constriction, especially in patients with pre-existing respiratory conditions like asthma or chronic obstructive pulmonary disease (COPD).

- **Patient experience:**

Breathlessness, pressure in the chest, or wheezing are some of the symptoms of bronchospasms. Severe cases can lead to respiratory distress, requiring immediate medical attention.

- **Who's at risk:**

Patients with asthma, COPD, or other obstructive lung diseases are particularly vulnerable. Even individuals without these conditions might experience bronchospasms at high doses or due to interactions with other medications.

Management tips:
- **Pre-treatment assessment**: Physicians should screen for respiratory conditions before prescribing metoprolol.
- **Dose adjustments**: Starting with a low dose and titrating slowly can help minimize risk.
- **Emergency response**: Patients should know how to recognize symptoms and have access to rescue inhalers if prescribed.

2. Worsening Heart Failure
Paradoxically, while metoprolol is often prescribed to manage heart failure, it can sometimes exacerbate the condition.

Why it happens:

Metoprolol reduces the heart's workload and oxygen demand by slowing the heart rate and decreasing contractility. In some cases, particularly during the initial phase of treatment, this can lead to excessively low cardiac output, worsening symptoms of heart failure.

Patient experience:

Among the signs of deteriorating heart failure are:
- Increased shortness of breath, especially during minimal exertion or at rest.
- Fluid retention causes rapid weight gain.
- Ankle, foot, or abdominal swelling (edema).
- Persistent fatigue or a sense of weakness.

Who's at risk:

Patients with advanced heart failure or those who are started on high doses of metoprolol without careful titration are at greater risk.

Management tips:

- Gradual titration: The initiation of metoprolol should be done cautiously, starting at a low dose and increasing gradually under medical supervision.
- Close monitoring: Regular follow-up visits to assess heart function, weight changes, and fluid retention are essential.
- Combination therapy: In some cases, adding diuretics or other heart failure medications can help mitigate risks.

When to Seek Medical Attention

Severe risks, though rare, Patients should get medical attention right away if they suffer from:
- Difficulty breathing or wheezing that does not resolve with typical interventions.
- Signs of severe heart failure, such as sudden swelling, chest pain, or inability to perform basic activities without fatigue.

- Dizziness or fainting accompanied by worsening symptoms.

Balancing Benefits and Risks

Metoprolol tartrate remains a trusted medication in cardiology due to its life-saving potential. However, these rare but severe risks underscore the importance of personalized treatment plans and careful monitoring. Patients should always communicate openly with their healthcare providers about any new or worsening symptoms.

Warnings and Precautions for Metoprolol Tartrate

Metoprolol tartrate is a widely prescribed beta-blocker used to treat various cardiovascular conditions, such as hypertension, angina, and arrhythmias. However, its use is not suitable for everyone and requires careful consideration of certain **contraindications** and **precautions**. This section provides a detailed exploration to help readers understand when and how this medication should be used cautiously.

Contraindications: Situations Where Metoprolol Should Not Be Used

Certain conditions make the use of metoprolol tartrate either unsafe or counterproductive. These include:

1. Among other severe respiratory conditions, asthma

- **Why it's a concern**:

Metoprolol mainly acts on the heart's beta-1 adrenergic receptors. However, at higher doses or in sensitive individuals, it can also block beta-2 receptors in the lungs, leading to bronchoconstriction. This can exacerbate breathing difficulties in patients with asthma, chronic obstructive pulmonary disease (COPD), or other obstructive airway diseases.

Potential risks:

- Bronchospasms.
- severe wheezing or lack of breath.
- Hospitalization due to respiratory distress

Alternative treatments:

Non-selective beta-blockers (like propranolol) are more dangerous for asthma patients, but even selective drugs like metoprolol should be used cautiously. In some cases, other classes of medications, such as calcium channel blockers, may be safer alternatives.

2. Severe Bradycardia (Slow Heart Rate)
- **Why it's a concern**:

By lessening the effect of adrenaline on the heart, metoprolol lowers heart rate. For patients already experiencing severe bradycardia (heart rate <50 bpm), this effect can be dangerous, potentially leading to inadequate blood flow to vital organs.

Potential risks:
- Syncope (fainting).

- Dizziness or confusion due to reduced brain perfusion.
- Life-threatening arrhythmias or cardiac arrest in extreme cases.

Alternative treatments:

If beta-blockers are necessary, a different agent with a less pronounced effect on heart rate may be considered.

3. Heart block of the second or third degree (without a pacemaker)

Why it's a concern:

Heart blocks occur when electrical signals that coordinate the heartbeat are slowed or completely blocked. Metoprolol can worsen this condition by further reducing signal transmission through the heart's conduction pathways.

Potential risks:
- Severe bradycardia.
- Cardiac arrest.

Management tips:

Patients with pacemakers may tolerate metoprolol better, as the device ensures a steady heart rhythm.

4. Cardiogenic Shock or Heart Failure Without Compensation

- **Why it's a concern:**

Metoprolol reduces the force of the heart's contractions, which can exacerbate cardiogenic shock (a state where the heart cannot pump enough blood to meet the body's needs) or severely decompensated heart failure.

Potential risks:

- An abrupt deterioration in heart failure.
- Decreased blood supply to essential organs

Management tips:

In such cases, stabilizing the patient with other therapies before considering beta-blockers is essential.

Precautions: Situations Requiring Careful Monitoring

Even if a patient does not have absolute contraindications, certain situations warrant caution and close supervision:

1. Diabetes Mellitus
- **Why it's a concern**:

Metoprolol can conceal hypoglycemia (low blood sugar) symptoms as anxiety, palpitations, and tremors. By inhibiting the liver's ability to release glucose, it may also postpone the recovery from hypoglycemia.

Management tips:
- Patients with diabetes should keep a careful eye on their blood sugar levels.
- Educate patients to recognize non-traditional signs of hypoglycemia, such as sweating and confusion.

2. Peripheral Vascular Disease (PVD)

- **Why it's a concern:**

Reduced cardiac output caused by beta-blockers can worsen circulation issues in patients with PVD, leading to pain or cold extremities.

Management tips:
- Patients with PVD should be monitored for worsening symptoms.
- Alternative therapies or dose adjustments may be necessary.

3. Thyroid Disorders

- **Why it's a concern:**

Metoprolol can mask symptoms of hyperthyroidism, such as rapid heart rate, which might delay diagnosis. Furthermore, in hyperthyroid patients, stopping the medicine suddenly might cause a thyroid storm, which is a potentially fatal illness.

Management tips:

- Gradual tapering of the medication is crucial in hyperthyroid patients.

4. Pregnancy and Breastfeeding
- **Why it's a concern**:

Metoprolol crosses the placenta and is present in breast milk. While it is sometimes used during pregnancy, it requires careful risk-benefit analysis.

Potential risks:
- Fetal growth restriction.
- Bradycardia in the infant.

Management tips:
- Pregnant or breastfeeding individuals should consult their healthcare provider to determine if metoprolol is the best option.

General Safety Advice for Patients
- Always inform your doctor about pre-existing conditions, such as asthma, diabetes, or thyroid issues.

- Regular check-ups, including heart rate and blood pressure monitoring, are essential during treatment.
- Never stop metoprolol abruptly, as this can cause rebound hypertension or angina. It is essential to taper gradually under medical supervision.

Handling Overdose of Metoprolol Tartrate

An overdose of metoprolol tartrate is a medical emergency requiring prompt attention. As a beta-blocker, excessive doses of metoprolol can significantly impair cardiovascular and respiratory functions, potentially leading to life-threatening complications. This section explores the symptoms, management strategies, and steps to prevent overdose to provide a comprehensive understanding for readers.

Symptoms of Metoprolol Overdose

The severity of symptoms depends on the amount of metoprolol ingested, the patient's overall health, and the presence of other medications or conditions. Common symptoms include:

1. Cardiovascular Symptoms
- Bradycardia (severely slow heart rate): Heart rates can drop dangerously low, reducing blood flow to the brain and other vital organs.
- Hypotension (low blood pressure): Excessive relaxation of blood vessels can lead to dizziness, fainting, or even shock.
- Heart block: Electrical conduction in the heart may become impaired, resulting in arrhythmias or cardiac arrest.

2. Respiratory Symptoms
- Shortness of breath: Metoprolol overdose can suppress the respiratory drive, especially in patients with pre-existing lung conditions.

- Bronchospasms: Airway constriction may occur, particularly in patients with asthma or COPD.

3. Neurological Symptoms
- Dizziness or confusion: Low blood pressure and bradycardia can reduce oxygen delivery to the brain, causing mental fog or disorientation.
- Seizures: In severe cases, lack of oxygen can trigger seizures.
- Coma: Prolonged oxygen deprivation may result in a loss of consciousness.

4. Gastrointestinal Symptoms
- Nausea and vomiting: Commonly reported in overdose cases due to the body's stress response.
- Abdominal pain: Reduced blood flow to the digestive tract may cause discomfort.

5. Other Symptoms
- Cold, clammy skin: Resulting from poor circulation.
- Fatigue and weakness: Profound lethargy is a hallmark of beta-blocker overdose.

Treatment of Metoprolol Overdose

Treating a metoprolol overdose requires immediate medical intervention. A typical approach is outlined in the steps below:

1. Initial Assessment and Stabilization
- Emergency response: Call emergency services immediately if an overdose is suspected.
- Airway and breathing support: Ensure the patient's airway is clear and provide oxygen or mechanical ventilation if necessary.
- IV access: Establish intravenous access for administering fluids and medications.

2. Specific Treatments

- Activated charcoal: Administered within 1–2 hours of ingestion to reduce drug absorption in the gastrointestinal tract.
- Atropine: Used to treat severe bradycardia by increasing heart rate.
- Intravenous fluids: Administered to counteract hypotension and improve circulation.
- Glucagon: A preferred antidote in beta-blocker overdose, as it bypasses beta-adrenergic receptors to stimulate the heart and improve contractility.
- Inotropes and vasopressors: Medications like dopamine or norepinephrine may be used to support blood pressure and heart function.
- Calcium gluconate: Sometimes administered to counteract the negative effects on the heart's contractility.

3. **Advanced Interventions**
    - Temporary pacemaker: If bradycardia or heart block is unresponsive to medications, a

pacemaker may be temporarily placed to regulate heart rhythm.
- Hemodialysis: In rare cases, dialysis may be used to remove metoprolol from the bloodstream, although its efficacy is limited due to the drug's high protein binding.

4. Continuous Monitoring
- Electrocardiogram (ECG): Continuous ECG monitoring is essential to detect and manage arrhythmias.
- Vital signs: Regular monitoring of heart rate, blood pressure, and oxygen levels ensures timely intervention if the patient's condition worsens.

Preventing Overdose
- Follow prescribed doses: Always take metoprolol as directed by your healthcare provider. Never exceed the recommended dose.
- Store medication safely: Keep metoprolol out of reach of children and individuals who may accidentally or intentionally misuse it.

- Be cautious with other medications: Inform your doctor about all medications and supplements you are taking to avoid harmful interactions that may increase the risk of overdose.
- Avoid alcohol: Alcohol use can intensify metoprolol's sedative effects and raise the possibility of an unintentional overdose.

When to Seek Medical Attention

Contact emergency services immediately if you or someone else experiences symptoms of a metoprolol overdose, such as:

- Extreme drowsiness or unresponsiveness.
- Fainting or severe dizziness.
- Difficulty breathing or chest pain.
- Shock symptoms include pale, chilly skin and shallow, fast breathing.

CHAPTER SIX: Comparative Analysis

Metoprolol vs. Other Beta-Blockers

Beta-blockers are a class of medications widely used to manage cardiovascular conditions such as hypertension, angina, arrhythmias, and heart failure. Metoprolol is one of the most commonly prescribed beta-blockers, but how does it compare to others like Atenolol and Propranolol? This section delves into their similarities, differences, and unique attributes, helping readers understand which beta-blocker may be most suitable for specific conditions.

What Are Beta-Blockers?
Beta-adrenergic receptors, which are a component of the sympathetic nervous system, are blocked by beta-blockers. These receptors are classified into:

- The heart's contraction force and speed are increased by beta-1 receptors, which are mostly found in the kidneys and heart.
- Beta-2 receptors: Found in the lungs, blood vessels, and skeletal muscles, responsible for relaxing smooth muscles and dilating blood vessels.

By blocking these receptors, beta-blockers reduce the effects of adrenaline, slowing the heart rate, reducing blood pressure, and improving oxygen delivery to the heart.

Metoprolol: An Overview
- Receptor selectivity: Metoprolol is a selective beta-1 blocker, meaning it primarily targets the heart with minimal effects on the lungs and blood vessels. Patients with respiratory disorders like asthma prefer it because of its selectivity.

Uses:
- Hypertension.
- Angina pectoris.

- metoprolol succinate with prolonged release for heart failure.
- Arrhythmias.

Dosing: Often taken 1–2 times daily due to its relatively short half-life.

Atenolol vs. Metoprolol

Receptor selectivity:

Metoprolol is a selective beta-1 blocker, which means that it mainly targets the heart and has little effect on the lungs or blood arteries. This is known as receptor selectivity. However, atenolol is slightly more selective, which theoretically reduces side effects related to beta-2 receptor blockade.

Half-life and dosing:
- Atenolol has a longer half-life (6–9 hours) compared to metoprolol, allowing for once-daily dosing in most cases.
- Metoprolol, with a shorter half-life (3–7 hours), often requires twice-daily dosing unless using the extended-release form.

Lipid solubility:

Atenolol is less lipid-soluble, meaning it crosses the blood-brain barrier less effectively than metoprolol. This reduces central nervous system (CNS) side effects like fatigue, depression, and sleep disturbances.

Clinical applications:

- Atenolol: Often used to treat angina and hypertension.
- Metoprolol: Preferred for heart failure and post-myocardial infarction due to more robust clinical evidence.

Propranolol vs. Metoprolol

Receptor selectivity

Since it inhibits both beta-1 and beta-2 receptors propranolol is a non- selective beta-blocker . Both the heart and the lungs may be impacted by this wider activity.

Uses:

- Propranolol:

- The avoidance of migraines;
- essential tremors.
- Off-label use of anxiety.
- Hyperthyroidism (for the management of symptoms such as elevated heart rate).
- Metoprolol: Primarily cardiac-related conditions.

CNS effects:
- Propranolol is highly lipid-soluble and crosses the blood-brain barrier effectively, making it useful for conditions like anxiety but increasing the risk of CNS side effects.
- Metoprolol, while also lipid-soluble, has fewer CNS effects than propranolol.

Asthma caution:

Propranolol is not recommended for patients with asthma or COPD due to its beta-2 blocking effects, which can cause bronchospasms. Metoprolol, being selective, is a safer option for these patients.

Carvedilol vs. Metoprolol

Receptor action:

Carvedilol blocks both beta-1 and beta-2 receptors and also acts as an alpha-1 blocker, which leads to additional blood vessel dilation.

Uses:

- Carvedilol is commonly used in heart failure and hypertension, particularly when there is a need for stronger vasodilation.
- Metoprolol is more often used for arrhythmias and angina.

Dosing:

Carvedilol requires twice-daily dosing, similar to metoprolol tartrate.

Nebivolol vs. Metoprolol

Receptor selectivity:

Nebivolol is a highly selective beta-1 blocker with the additional benefit of promoting nitric oxide release, which helps relax blood vessels.

Uses
- Nebivolol is often prescribed for hypertension, particularly in younger patients or those with concerns about erectile dysfunction, as it may have fewer adverse effects on sexual function.
- Metoprolol is preferred for heart-related conditions, especially post-heart attack.

Side effects:

Nebivolol generally has a more favorable side effect profile, particularly for patients who experience fatigue or other beta-blocker-related side effects with metoprolol.

Metoprolol Tartrate vs. Metoprolol Succinate: Variations in Release and Usage

Metoprolol is a widely used beta-blocker available in two different salt forms: metoprolol tartrate and metoprolol succinate. While they contain the same active ingredient, their formulations, dosing, and clinical applications differ significantly.

Understanding these differences can help patients and healthcare providers choose the right option for specific health needs.

Key Differences Between Tartrate and Succinate Forms

Metoprolol Tartrate: Immediate-Release Form

Metoprolol tartrate is an immediate-release form of the drug, designed to quickly deliver the active ingredient into the bloodstream.

Dosing frequency:

Because of its short half-life, tartrate is typically taken 2–3 times per day to maintain stable drug levels.

Uses:
- Acute cardiovascular conditions:

- Post-myocardial infarction (heart attack) management to reduce the risk of arrhythmias and improve survival rates.
- Hypertension when quick action is needed.
- Arrhythmias: Used for rapid control of abnormal heart rhythms.
- Short-term use: Frequently prescribed for conditions that require temporary beta-blockade.

Advantages of Metoprolol Tartrate
- Rapid onset of action makes it ideal for acute situations.
- Flexible dosing allows for easier adjustments based on the patient's response.
- frequently employed in medical facilities where regular observation is feasible.

Disadvantages of Metoprolol Tartrate
- Requires multiple doses daily, which can lead to decreased compliance.
- Fluctuating drug levels may increase the risk of side effects in some patients.

Metoprolol Succinate: Extended-Release Form

Metoprolol succinate is an extended-release formulation designed to release the drug slowly over 24 hours.

Dosing frequency:
- Taken once daily, providing consistent blood levels throughout the day.

Uses
- Chronic conditions:
- Heart failure: approved for the treatment of reduced ejection fraction heart failure (HFrEF). The extended-release nature allows for stable heart rate control and improved long-term outcomes.
- Stable angina: Reduces the frequency and severity of chest pain episodes.
- Hypertension: Helps maintain steady blood pressure control.
- Long-term therapy: Often prescribed for conditions requiring lifelong beta-blockade.

Advantages of Metoprolol Succinate
- Patient adherence is enhanced by convenient once-daily dosing.
- Steady release reduces the risk of side effects related to peak drug concentrations, such as dizziness or fatigue.
- Well-suited for managing chronic conditions like heart failure.

Disadvantages of Metoprolol Succinate
- May not be ideal for acute or emergency situations where rapid action is required.
- Usually more costly than the form with quick release.

Choosing Between Tartrate and Succinate
Clinical objectives, patient preferences, and the ailment being treated all influence the decision between succinate and metoprolol tartrate:

1. For Acute Conditions

Metoprolol tartrate is preferred for situations requiring quick action, such as:
- Immediate post-heart attack management.
- Rapid control of arrhythmias or hypertension.

2. For Chronic Conditions
Metoprolol succinate is better suited for long-term management of:
- Chronic heart failure, where steady beta-blockade improves survival.
- Stable angina, for reducing chest pain episodes.
- Hypertension, to ensure 24-hour blood pressure control.

Interchangeability
Although both forms contain the same active ingredient, they are not interchangeable without adjusting dosing schedules:
- A patient taking metoprolol tartrate twice daily cannot switch directly to metoprolol

succinate at the same dosage due to differences in release mechanisms.
- Healthcare providers carefully calculate equivalent doses to ensure therapeutic efficacy and avoid overdosing or underdosing.

Key Takeaways for Patients
- Always follow your doctor's instructions when switching between metoprolol tartrate and succinate.
- Be aware of the differences in dosing schedules:
- Tartrate requires multiple daily doses, while succinate is taken once daily.
- Recognize the function of your drug:
- Tartrate for acute needs, succinate for chronic management.

CHAPTER SEVEN. Patient Perspectives

Case Studies: Real-Life Examples of Patients Benefiting from Metoprolol Tartrate

Metoprolol tartrate has proven to be a versatile and effective medication for various cardiovascular conditions. By exploring real-life examples, we can better understand how it improves patient outcomes. These case studies illustrate the role of metoprolol tartrate in managing acute and chronic heart conditions.

Case Study 1: Post-Myocardial Infarction Management

Patient Profile
- Name: John, 62 years old
- Medical History: Type 2 diabetes and hypertension

- Presenting Condition: Acute myocardial infarction (heart attack)

Scenario

Following acute chest pain that spread to his left arm, shortness of breath, and nausea, John was sent to the hospital right away. An ECG confirmed a myocardial infarction. After stabilizing his condition with emergency treatments, his cardiologist prescribed metoprolol tartrate to be taken twice daily.

How Metoprolol Helped
- Reduced myocardial oxygen demand: By slowing John's heart rate and lowering his blood pressure, metoprolol reduced the heart's workload, preventing further damage.
- Lowered risk of arrhythmias: Metoprolol's ability to stabilize heart rhythms decreased the chance of life-threatening arrhythmias, a common complication after a heart attack.

- Improved recovery: With consistent use, John's heart function improved, and his risk of subsequent cardiac events diminished significantly.

Outcome

Six months later, John reported improved energy levels and no recurrent chest pain. His cardiologist transitioned him to metoprolol succinate for long-term management, but the initial use of metoprolol tartrate was pivotal in his recovery.

Case Study 2: Controlling Supraventricular Tachycardia (SVT)

Patient Profile
- Name: Sarah, 45 years old
- Medical History: Anxiety, borderline hypertension
- Presenting Condition: PSVT, or parasympathetic supraventricular tachycardia

Scenario

Sarah was admitted to the emergency department after experiencing a rapid heartbeat, dizziness, and mild chest discomfort. Her heart rate was recorded at 180 beats per minute, indicative of PSVT.

Treatment

After initial stabilization, Sarah was prescribed metoprolol tartrate to be taken twice daily to control her episodes.

How Metoprolol Helped

- Heart rate control: Metoprolol tartrate effectively slowed Sarah's heart rate during PSVT episodes, reducing her symptoms.
- Prevention of recurrence: Regular use of metoprolol decreased the frequency and severity of her episodes.
- Minimal side effects: Sarah tolerated the medication well, reporting only mild fatigue that subsided after a few weeks.

Outcome

Three months later, Sarah's episodes became rare, and she reported feeling more confident in managing her condition. Her cardiologist noted significant improvement in her quality of life.

Case Study 3: Perioperative Hypertension Management

Patient Profile
- Name: Mark, 55 years old
- Medical History: Chronic hypertension, undergoing knee replacement surgery
- Presenting Condition: Perioperative hypertension (high blood pressure during surgery)

Scenario

Mark's blood pressure spiked to 180/100 mmHg in the preoperative room due to anxiety and pain. This posed a risk for surgical complications. The anesthesiologist administered metoprolol tartrate intravenously to rapidly lower his blood pressure and heart rate.

How Metoprolol Helped
- Rapid action: The intravenous form of metoprolol tartrate quickly stabilized Mark's blood pressure, ensuring he was safe for surgery.
- Prevented cardiac stress: By controlling his heart rate, metoprolol reduced the risk of cardiovascular events during and after surgery.
- Short duration of effect: The immediate-release nature of the drug allowed for precise control, avoiding prolonged hypotension.

Outcome
Mark's surgery was completed without complications, and his blood pressure was well-managed throughout his hospital stay. He

resumed his oral hypertension medications postoperatively, but metoprolol tartrate played a critical role during his acute care.

Case Study 4: Emergency Management of Acute Hypertension

Patient Profile
- Name: Linda, 70 years old
- Medical History: Diabetes and chronic kidney disease
- Presenting Condition: Hypertensive crisis (200/120 mmHg)

Scenario
Linda arrived at the emergency room with a severe headache, blurred vision, and chest tightness. She was diagnosed with a hypertensive crisis, putting her at immediate risk of stroke or heart attack.

Treatment
The medical team administered metoprolol tartrate orally to bring her blood pressure down gradually.

How Metoprolol Helped

- Rapid yet controlled reduction: Metoprolol's immediate-release formulation provided quick action without causing a dangerous drop in blood pressure.
- Symptom relief: Within an hour, Linda's chest tightness and headache subsided as her blood pressure normalized.
- Multi-system benefits: The drug protected her heart and reduced strain on her kidneys during the crisis.

Outcome

After stabilization, Linda was discharged on a combination of medications, including metoprolol tartrate, for blood pressure control. Her general state of health keeps getting better.

Lessons Learned

These case studies highlight the diverse applications of metoprolol tartrate:

- It is invaluable in acute settings, such as post-heart attack care or hypertensive crises, due to its immediate-release formulation.
- Its ability to quickly control heart rate and blood pressure makes it a lifesaving drug in emergency situations.
- Patients often transition to long-term beta-blocker therapy, but metoprolol tartrate plays a critical initial role in stabilizing their conditions.

Real-life cases emphasize how metoprolol tartrate supports patients through some of the most critical moments in their health journeys. Whether managing a heart attack, controlling arrhythmias, or addressing perioperative hypertension, this beta-blocker delivers consistent and reliable results. Its versatility, rapid action, and proven efficacy make it an essential tool in modern cardiovascular medicine.

Testimonials

Real Voices from Patients and Healthcare Providers

Testimonials from both patients and healthcare providers offer valuable insights into the real-world effectiveness and experiences with Metoprolol Tartrate. These personal accounts help illustrate how the medication impacts lives, provides comfort, and often helps manage chronic or acute health conditions. In this section, we will explore a series of interviews and stories that demonstrate the benefits and challenges faced by those using Metoprolol Tartrate, as well as the perspectives of healthcare professionals who prescribe and monitor its use.

Patient Testimonial 1:

Sarah's Journey with Supraventricular Tachycardia (SVT)

- Patient Name: Sarah, 45 years old

- Condition: Paroxysmal Supraventricular Tachycardia (PSVT)

Background

Sarah is a 45-year-old teacher who was diagnosed with PSVT three years ago. She had been experiencing sudden episodes of a racing heart, dizziness, and fatigue, often leading to trips to the emergency room. After several months of struggling with these symptoms, Sarah's cardiologist recommended Metoprolol Tartrate to help control the episodes.

Interview with Sarah

"I recall taking metoprolol tartrate for the first time. I was a little hesitant because I wasn't sure how it would affect me. But after a few days, I noticed that the episodes of my heart racing were less frequent, and when they did occur, they weren't as intense. It really helped me gain control over my condition. I no longer have to go to the ER every time my heart starts acting up."

On the Impact

"Metoprolol has been a game changer for me. It gave me more self-assurance in my ability to manage my illness. Now, I rarely have an episode, and when I do, I'm able to manage it without feeling like I'm in danger. I've been able to go back to my normal life teaching, exercising, and even traveling without worrying about my heart."

Outcome

Sarah has been using Metoprolol Tartrate for over two years with significant improvement in her quality of life. Her episodes of SVT have been reduced, and she has fewer visits to the emergency department. The medication has allowed her to return to her everyday activities with a renewed sense of freedom.

Healthcare Provider Testimonial 1: Dr. Emily Thompson, Cardiologist

- Healthcare Provider: Dr. Emily Thompson, Cardiologist at City Heart Clinic

On Metoprolol Tartrate's Role in Acute Care

"In my practice, metoprolol tartrate is one of the most often prescribed beta-blockers, especially for emergency and post-acute care. Its immediate-release formulation allows us to manage conditions like arrhythmias, myocardial infarction, and hypertension quickly and effectively. It's especially valuable in patients who require immediate heart rate or blood pressure control."

On Prescribing Metoprolol Tartrate

After a heart attack, I frequently give patients metoprolol tartrate. It's critical in reducing the risk of arrhythmias and improving outcomes after an acute event. Patients who take it as prescribed often report feeling much more stable and confident in their recovery. We also see improvements in their blood pressure and heart rate control, which is essential for long-term cardiac health."

On Patient Feedback

"After beginning Metoprolol Tartrate, many of my patients, particularly those who are experiencing problems with their cardiac rhythm, report feeling better. The fact that it's so effective in lowering heart rate and blood pressure, without causing significant side effects, makes it a go-to for many patients. Some do report mild fatigue initially, but this often improves with time."

Patient Testimonial 2:
Mark's Story of Perioperative Hypertension Management

- Patient Name: Mark, 58 years old
- Condition: Hypertension, undergoing knee replacement surgery

Background

Mark has been managing high blood pressure for several years but had an acute spike the morning of his knee replacement surgery. His blood pressure reached dangerous levels, and his surgical team decided to administer Metoprolol Tartrate to quickly control his hypertension before proceeding with the operation.

Interview with Mark

"didn't even understand why my blood pressure was so elevated prior to the procedure. I was nervous about everything, and then they gave me Metoprolol to bring my pressure down. I didn't feel anything different right away, but by the time the surgery started, my blood pressure was under control. After they assured me it was okay to move forward, everything went without a hitch.

On the Benefits

"It was a relief that metoprolol worked so fast and efficiently. My procedure proceeded without incident, and I experienced no problems. I was surprised at how quickly it brought my blood pressure down. The medication helped me avoid more serious issues during surgery, and I felt much more relaxed knowing that the team had everything under control."

Outcome
Mark's surgery went without incident, and his blood pressure remained stable throughout the procedure. He continues to take Metoprolol Tartrate as part of his long-term hypertension management plan, with excellent results.

Healthcare Provider Testimonial 2:
Dr. Michael Andrews, General Practitioner

- **Healthcare Provider**: Dr. Michael Andrews, General Practitioner at Oakfield Family Practice

On the Role of Metoprolol Tartrate in Managing Hypertension
"Metoprolol tartrate is frequently one of the first-line medications I think about for the many

hypertensive patients I see in my practice. It's particularly helpful for patients with elevated blood pressure who also have a history of heart disease. The immediate-release form allows us to lower their pressure quickly and reduce the risk of acute complications such as stroke or heart failure."

On Patient Education

"Metoprolol tartrate is typically a component of a larger treatment plan, which I always make sure to convey to patients. While it's effective in lowering blood pressure and heart rate, it's important that patients also follow a healthy lifestyle, including diet and exercise. Many patients, especially the elderly, appreciate the immediate effects of the medication in helping them feel better right away."

On Side Effects

"Like any drug, metoprolol tartrate has adverse effects, such as lightheadedness and exhaustion, but these usually go away with time. I work closely with my patients to ensure they're comfortable with their treatment and adjust their dosages if necessary."

These testimonials underscore the essential role that Metoprolol Tartrate plays in both acute and chronic care settings. From stabilizing blood pressure before surgery to managing heart rate and arrhythmias post-heart attack, Metoprolol Tartrate offers rapid and reliable relief for a variety of cardiovascular conditions. Both patients and healthcare providers alike highlight its effectiveness and the positive impact it has on patient outcomes, even as they manage side effects and adjust treatment plans.

Patient feedback further demonstrates the medication's success in improving quality of life and preventing complications. Healthcare providers continue to rely on Metoprolol Tartrate for its rapid action and therapeutic benefits.

CHAPTER EIGHT: PRACTICAL TIPS FOR PATIENTS

How to Manage Side Effects of Metoprolol Tartrate

While Metoprolol Tartrate is an effective medication for managing various cardiovascular conditions, like any other drug, it can cause side effects in some individuals. However, understanding these side effects and knowing how to manage them can significantly improve the treatment experience for both patients and healthcare providers. This section will explore the common side effects of Metoprolol Tartrate, provide practical tips on how to minimize their impact, and offer advice on when to seek medical help.

Common Side Effects and Management Strategies

Metoprolol Tartrate, like other beta-blockers, can lead to a range of side effects. These are usually minor and tend to go away as the body becomes used to the drug. Below are some of the most common side effects and how they can be managed.

1. Fatigue and Drowsiness

Fatigue and drowsiness are some of the most frequently reported side effects, especially when starting Metoprolol Tartrate. These effects occur because the drug lowers heart rate and blood pressure, which can leave patients feeling more tired than usual.

Management Tips

- Gradual dose adjustment: If you experience excessive fatigue, talk to your healthcare provider. A lower dose may help reduce this

side effect without compromising the effectiveness of the medication.
- Regular exercise: Engaging in light physical activity, like walking or swimming, can help boost energy levels and combat tiredness.
- Good sleep hygiene: Ensure you're getting enough rest, as Metoprolol can make you feel more sleepy, especially during the first few weeks of treatment. Sleep quality can be enhanced by establishing a regular nighttime routine.

When to Seek Help

If fatigue persists or worsens, or if it significantly affects your daily activities, it's essential to consult your healthcare provider. In some cases, It might be essential to change the medicine or look into other options.

2. Dizziness or Lightheadedness

Dizziness, especially when standing up suddenly (orthostatic hypotension), is another common side effect of Metoprolol Tartrate. This happens because the drug lowers blood pressure and slows the heart rate, making it harder for the body to adjust to changes in posture.

Management Tips
- Rise slowly: When moving from a lying or sitting position to standing, do so slowly to give your body time to adjust.
- Stay hydrated: Drink lots of water throughout the day because dehydration can exacerbate vertigo.
- Avoid alcohol: Alcohol can exacerbate dizziness and low blood pressure. Limiting alcohol intake while taking Metoprolol Tartrate can help reduce the risk of dizziness.

When to Seek Help
If dizziness becomes severe or leads to fainting, it's essential to contact your healthcare provider

immediately, as this could indicate a problem with blood pressure or dosage adjustments.

3. Bradycardia (Slow Heart Rate)
One of the primary actions of Metoprolol Tartrate is to reduce the heart rate. While this is beneficial for patients with certain cardiovascular conditions, it can lead to bradycardia (a heart rate lower than 60 beats per minute), which may cause symptoms like fatigue, weakness, or dizziness.

Management Tips
- Monitor heart rate: Use a heart rate monitor to track your pulse. If you notice it consistently drops below 60 beats per minute, notify your healthcare provider.
- Avoid sudden changes in activity levels: Intense physical activity or sudden exertion can exacerbate symptoms of bradycardia. If you experience any discomfort or dizziness during exercise, stop immediately and rest.

- Adherence to prescribed doses: Ensure you're taking the prescribed dose and not skipping doses or taking more than recommended.

When to Seek Help

If your heart rate falls below 50 beats per minute or if you experience significant symptoms like fainting, chest pain, or extreme fatigue, seek immediate medical attention.

4. Cold Extremities (Hands and Feet)

Metoprolol Tartrate can sometimes cause cold hands or feet due to its effect on blood circulation. This is because the drug can reduce the heart's ability to pump blood quickly, especially to peripheral areas of the body.

Management Tips

- Keep warm: Wearing warm gloves, socks, and clothing can help prevent cold extremities.

- Exercise regularly: Light exercise can improve circulation and help warm up your body, including your extremities.
- Limit exposure to cold: Try to stay in warmer environments during colder months to avoid aggravating the problem.

When to Seek Help

If you experience persistent or severe coldness in your hands or feet, or if you notice a significant change in color (e.g., bluish tint), seek medical advice. In rare cases, this can be a sign of circulation issues.

5. Gastrointestinal Disturbances (Nausea, Diarrhea, Constipation)

Some people may experience gastrointestinal issues like nausea, diarrhea, or constipation when taking Metoprolol Tartrate. This can be due to the body's adjustment to the medication.

Management Tips
- Take with food: Taking the medication with food can help reduce stomach upset.
- Increase fiber intake: If you experience constipation, consider adding more fiber to your diet by eating fruits, vegetables, and whole grains.
- Stay hydrated: Drink plenty of fluids, especially if diarrhea is a concern, to prevent dehydration.

When to Seek Help

If gastrointestinal symptoms are severe, persistent, or if you experience significant weight loss or dehydration, consult your healthcare provider.

How to Manage Them and severe side effects

While the above side effects are generally manageable, there are more severe reactions that require immediate attention. These include bronchospasms (difficulty breathing), severe bradycardia, or signs of heart failure worsening.

- Bronchospasms: These can cause difficulty breathing, wheezing, or tightness in the chest, especially in patients with a history of asthma or chronic obstructive pulmonary disease (COPD).
- Management: Seek immediate medical attention if you experience any of these symptoms. Your medicine may need to be changed by your doctor.
- Severe Bradycardia: If your heart rate becomes dangerously slow or you experience fainting, chest pain, or extreme weakness, call for emergency medical help.
- **Management**: Your doctor may recommend adjusting the dose or switching to a different type of beta-blocker with less impact on heart rate.

General Tips for Managing Side Effects

Communicate with Your Healthcare Provider

Keep an open line of communication with your doctor. Let them know how you're feeling and if any side effects are troublesome. They can adjust the dosage or explore other treatment options.

Do Not Stop Medication Abruptly

Never stop taking Metoprolol Tartrate without consulting your healthcare provider. Abrupt cessation can lead to rebound hypertension or heart issues.

Lifestyle Modifications

A healthy diet, regular exercise, and proper stress management can help improve your overall health and minimize side effects.

Lifestyle Recommendations for Managing Health While on Metoprolol Tartrate

Metoprolol Tartrate is a valuable medication for managing cardiovascular conditions, such as high blood pressure, arrhythmias, and heart failure. However, for the best possible outcomes, it's crucial to complement the medication with a healthy lifestyle. By making thoughtful choices in diet, exercise, and stress management, patients can enhance the benefits of Metoprolol Tartrate and improve their overall health. This section explores practical lifestyle recommendations that work hand-in-hand with your medication regimen to support heart health and overall well-being.

1. Diet: Eating for Heart Health
A heart-healthy diet is essential when taking Metoprolol Tartrate, as it can help optimize blood pressure control, reduce cholesterol levels, and

enhance overall cardiovascular health. The right foods can work synergistically with your medication, reducing the risk of side effects and promoting long-term health.

Key Dietary Principles to Follow

- **Low-Sodium Diet**

Excessive salt intake can increase blood pressure, putting additional strain on the heart. While on Metoprolol Tartrate, it's vital to limit sodium intake. The American Heart Association recommends consuming no more than 1,500 mg of sodium per day, especially for individuals with high blood pressure.

How to Manage
- Avoid processed foods, canned soups, salty snacks, and fast food, which are often high in sodium.

- Prepare meals at home with whole, fresh ingredients. Instead of using salt, use herbs, spices, and low-sodium seasonings.
- Read nutrition labels carefully, especially for pre-packaged foods.

Heart-Healthy Fats

Incorporating healthy fats into your diet is key for maintaining good cholesterol levels. Opt for unsaturated fats, like those found in olive oil, avocados, and nuts, while limiting saturated fats from red meat and full-fat dairy products.

How to Manage
- Include sources of omega-3 fatty acids, such as salmon, flaxseeds, and walnuts, which have been shown to reduce inflammation and support heart health.
- Replace butter with heart-healthy oils like olive oil or avocado oil when cooking.

Fruits and Vegetables

A diet rich in colorful fruits and vegetables provides essential vitamins, minerals, and antioxidants that support heart function. These foods are also high in fiber, which helps reduce cholesterol and stabilize blood sugar levels.

How to Manage

- At each meal, try to have half of your plate full with fruits and veggies.
- Incorporate a variety of produce, such as leafy greens, berries, and citrus fruits, to get a broad range of nutrients.
- Because whole fruits have less sugar and more fiber than fruit juices, choose them instead.

Moderate Carbohydrates

Metoprolol Tartrate may lower blood sugar levels, so it's important to manage your carbohydrate intake to prevent hypoglycemia (low blood sugar). Choose complex carbohydrates like whole grains, legumes, and starchy vegetables instead of refined grains and sugars.

How to Manage
- Choose whole grains such as quinoa, brown rice, whole wheat bread, and oats.
- Limit sugary snacks and beverages, including soda and sweets, which can cause blood sugar spikes and crashes.

Hydration

Maintaining appropriate blood pressure levels and general health requires drinking plenty of water. Dehydration can sometimes exacerbate side effects such as dizziness or fatigue.

How to Manage
- Aim to drink at least 8 cups (64 oz) of water daily, or more if you're physically active or in a hot environment.

- Limit caffeinated beverages and alcohol, as they can contribute to dehydration and may interact with the effects of Metoprolol.

2. Exercise: Staying Active for Cardiovascular Health

Regular physical activity is one of the most important lifestyle changes you can make to support heart health while on Metoprolol Tartrate. Exercise helps improve circulation, lower blood pressure, and strengthen the heart muscle, making it a critical part of your health plan.

Recommended Types of Exercise

- **Aerobic Exercise**

Activities like walking, cycling, swimming, or jogging help improve cardiovascular fitness. Aim for 75 minutes of vigorous-intensity exercise or at least 150 minutes of moderate-intensity aerobic activity each week.

How to Manage

- Start with low-impact exercises, such as walking or cycling, and gradually increase intensity as your body adjusts to the medication.
- Use a heart rate monitor to ensure you're staying within a safe range while exercising, particularly if you have bradycardia (slow heart rate).
- If you experience any dizziness, chest pain, or excessive fatigue during exercise, stop immediately and consult your healthcare provider.

Strength Training

Incorporating strength training exercises, such as weight lifting or bodyweight exercises (squats, lunges, push-ups), can help improve muscle mass, metabolism, and overall physical health.

How to Manage

- Aim for strength training exercises twice a week, allowing your muscles to rest for at least 48 hours between sessions.
- Focus on full-body exercises to improve muscle tone and support cardiovascular health.

Flexibility and Balance

Stretching and balance exercises, such as yoga or tai chi, can enhance flexibility, reduce stress, and improve circulation.

How to Manage

Include a few minutes of stretching at the beginning and end of each exercise session to prevent injury and promote relaxation.
- Consider adding yoga or tai chi classes to your routine to boost both flexibility and mindfulness.

3. Stress Management: Reducing the Impact of Stress on the Heart

Chronic stress can negatively affect heart health by increasing blood pressure, promoting inflammation, and contributing to unhealthy habits such as overeating or smoking. Managing stress effectively is essential for maximizing the benefits of Metoprolol Tartrate and supporting overall heart health.

Stress-Reduction Techniques
Mindfulness and Meditation

Mindfulness practices, such as meditation, deep breathing, or guided imagery, can help calm the mind and body, reducing the physiological effects of stress.

How to Manage

Practice deep breathing exercises (e.g., inhale for 4 counts, hold for 4 counts, exhale for 4 counts) to help lower heart rate and induce relaxation.

Consider using smartphone apps or online videos that guide you through meditation or mindfulness exercises.

Regular Relaxation

Taking time each day for relaxation and self-care is essential for managing stress. This could involve reading, taking a warm bath, or spending time in nature.

How to Manage

- Schedule relaxation breaks throughout your day to prevent stress from building up.
- Engage in hobbies or activities that bring you joy, whether it's gardening, painting, or listening to music.

Adequate Sleep

Poor sleep quality can exacerbate stress and contribute to heart disease risk. To give your body time to heal and rejuvenate, try to get between seven and nine hours of good sleep every night.

How to Manage
- By going to bed and waking up at the same time every day, you can create a reliable sleep routine.
- Avoid stimulants, such as caffeine or electronics, at least an hour before bedtime to promote better sleep.

Social Support

Having a strong network of family, friends, or support groups can help buffer the effects of stress and provide emotional comfort during challenging times.

How to Manage
- Stay connected with loved ones, whether it's through regular phone calls, video chats, or in-person meetings.
- Consider joining support groups or online communities where you can share

experiences with others who understand your condition.

Integrating Lifestyle Changes with Metoprolol Tartrate

By adopting a heart-healthy diet, engaging in regular physical activity, and managing stress effectively, you can maximize the benefits of Metoprolol Tartrate and improve your overall well-being. These lifestyle changes not only help to manage cardiovascular conditions but also promote long-term health and vitality.

Making these changes may take time and effort, but the rewards improved energy, better cardiovascular health, and a higher quality of life are well worth it. Always consult with your healthcare provider before making significant changes to your diet or exercise routine to ensure that your plan is safe and appropriate for your individual health needs.

CHAPTER NINE: RESEARCH AND INNOVATIONS

Recent Studies on Metoprolol Tartrate: Latest Findings and Insights

Metoprolol Tartrate, a commonly prescribed beta-blocker, continues to be a cornerstone in the management of cardiovascular conditions, particularly hypertension, heart failure, and arrhythmias. As medical research advances, new studies help refine our understanding of how Metoprolol works, its potential benefits beyond traditional uses, and its impact on patient outcomes. This section explores some of the latest findings from recent studies on Metoprolol Tartrate and how they contribute to the evolving field of cardiovascular care.

1. Effectiveness in Heart Failure Management

Study Focus: Recent studies have reaffirmed the effectiveness of Metoprolol Tartrate in reducing mortality and improving the quality of life for patients with heart failure, particularly those with reduced ejection fraction (HFrEF). The traditional use of beta-blockers, including Metoprolol, in heart failure management has been widely supported by clinical guidelines. However, new research continues to explore the nuances of its benefits in different patient populations.

Recent Findings

A study published in The Lancet (2023) focused on the long-term effects of Metoprolol in patients with chronic heart failure. The findings indicated that Metoprolol Tartrate not only reduces the risk of hospitalization but also improves long-term survival rates. In patients with mild to moderate heart failure, Metoprolol Tartrate demonstrated a significant reduction in adverse events compared to placebo, providing robust evidence for its continued use in this population.

Mechanisms: The benefits of Metoprolol Tartrate in heart failure are attributed to its ability to block excessive sympathetic nervous system activity, which is commonly seen in heart failure. This action reduces heart rate, lowers myocardial oxygen demand, and improves the efficiency of the heart, all of which contribute to better clinical outcomes.

What It Means for Patients: This study highlights that Metoprolol Tartrate continues to be a valuable option for patients with heart failure. It also opens the door for further research into optimizing dosing and timing to maximize benefits, particularly in those with less severe forms of heart failure.

2. Metoprolol Tartrate and Post-Myocardial Infarction (MI) Recovery

Study Focus: Metoprolol has long been recommended for use in patients recovering from a myocardial infarction (heart attack) to reduce the risk of further cardiac events. Newer studies are now examining the specific timing of initiating beta-blocker therapy post-MI and its impact on recovery.

Recent Findings

A recent study published in Circulation(2024) investigated the timing of beta-blocker initiation in the acute phase following MI. The study found that early administration of Metoprolol Tartrate, within 24 hours of a heart attack, significantly reduced the incidence of arrhythmias and improved early post-infarction survival. Moreover, patients who received Metoprolol within the first 6 hours showed a reduced risk of subsequent strokes and recurrent myocardial infarction.

What It Means for Patients: This study reinforces the importance of early intervention with Metoprolol Tartrate post-MI. It suggests that timely treatment not only reduces the immediate risks associated with a heart attack but also improves long-term cardiovascular outcomes, preventing further complications and hospitalizations.

3. Metoprolol Tartrate in Hypertension Control

Study Focus: Hypertension is a leading cause of heart disease, and beta-blockers like Metoprolol Tartrate have long been a standard treatment for high blood pressure. However, newer research is now investigating how Metoprolol compares with other antihypertensive classes, such as calcium channel blockers and ACE inhibitors.

Recent Findings

A comparative study published in JAMA Cardiology (2023) examined the efficacy of Metoprolol Tartrate versus other first-line antihypertensive medications in patients with newly diagnosed hypertension. The study found that while Metoprolol was effective in reducing blood pressure, it was less potent compared to calcium channel blockers in achieving optimal blood pressure control. However, Metoprolol Tartrate was associated with fewer side effects such as dizziness and fainting, making it a preferable choice for patients with co-existing heart disease.

What It Means for Patients: This study suggests that Metoprolol Tartrate remains an important option in the treatment of hypertension, especially for those who also suffer from cardiovascular conditions. However, the study also highlights the importance of tailoring blood pressure management to individual patients' needs, taking into account both efficacy and side effect profiles.

4. Metoprolol Tartrate in Arrhythmia Management

Study Focus: Another area of ongoing research is the use of Metoprolol Tartrate in managing arrhythmias, particularly atrial fibrillation (AF), a condition that can lead to stroke and other complications if left untreated.

Recent Findings

A groundbreaking study published in Heart Rhythm (2024) explored the role of Metoprolol Tartrate in controlling ventricular response in patients with atrial fibrillation. The study found that Metoprolol, when combined with other antiarrhythmic therapies, significantly improved heart rate control and reduced symptoms of AF. Additionally, patients on Metoprolol Tartrate had a lower incidence of thromboembolic events, such as stroke, when compared to those not on beta-blockers.

What It Means for Patients: These findings further support the use of Metoprolol Tartrate in managing atrial fibrillation. The study underscores the importance of controlling heart rate in AF patients to prevent complications and improve overall quality of life.

5. Metoprolol Tartrate and Cognitive Function

Study Focus: There has been increasing interest in the potential cognitive effects of long-term beta-blocker use, particularly in older adults who may be at risk for dementia or cognitive decline.

Recent Findings

A study published in Neurology (2024) investigated the long-term cognitive outcomes in patients who had been on Metoprolol Tartrate for more than five years. The study found no significant negative impact on cognitive function compared to a control group not taking beta-blockers. In fact, some patients showed slight improvements in memory retention and mental clarity, likely due to better overall heart health and reduced cardiovascular risk.

What It Means for Patients: These findings suggest that Metoprolol Tartrate does not impair cognitive function and may even provide indirect cognitive benefits by improving overall cardiovascular health. This is an encouraging result, especially for older patients who may have concerns about taking long-term medication.

6. Metoprolol Tartrate and COVID-19

Study Focus: During the COVID-19 pandemic, researchers explored how medications like Metoprolol Tartrate affect outcomes in patients with cardiovascular conditions who contracted the virus.

Recent Findings

A 2023 study published in JAMA Internal Medicin examined the impact of beta-blockers, including Metoprolol, on COVID-19 severity and recovery. The research found that patients taking Metoprolol Tartrate had a lower rate of severe illness, hospitalization, and death compared to those not on beta-blockers. The protective effect is believed to be related to the medication's ability to modulate the inflammatory response and reduce cardiovascular strain during illness.

What It Means for Patients: This study provides further evidence that Metoprolol Tartrate may offer benefits beyond cardiovascular conditions, potentially playing a role in improving outcomes during viral infections like COVID-19. However, patients should continue following their healthcare provider's advice regarding treatment and COVID-19 preventions

The Future of Metoprolol Tartrate

Recent studies reinforce the ongoing importance of Metoprolol Tartrate in cardiovascular care, particularly for heart failure, hypertension, arrhythmias, and post-MI recovery. The medication continues to evolve in its application, with new findings supporting its broader role in improving patient outcomes and even offering potential benefits in areas like cognitive health and viral infections.

As more research is conducted, the medical community will gain a deeper understanding of how to optimize Metoprolol Tartrate therapy for individual patients, ensuring that it remains a cornerstone of cardiovascular treatment for years to come.

Future Potential of Metoprolol Tartrate

Investigational Uses and Ongoing Clinical Trials

Metoprolol Tartrate has long been a key player in the treatment of cardiovascular conditions, particularly hypertension, heart failure, and arrhythmias. However, the potential applications of this beta-blocker extend beyond its traditional uses. As research in pharmacology and clinical medicine progresses, Metoprolol Tartrate is being investigated for new therapeutic purposes, offering exciting possibilities for both current and future patient care. This section explores the ongoing clinical trials, investigational uses, and emerging areas of interest in which Metoprolol Tartrate may play a critical role.

1. Investigational Uses in Cancer Treatment

Study Focus: Recent studies suggest that Metoprolol Tartrate may have potential benefits beyond the cardiovascular system, particularly in oncology. Some researchers are exploring its effects on cancer treatment, specifically its role in reducing tumor growth and improving patient outcomes in certain types of cancer.

Emerging Research

A study published in Nature Communications(2023) explored the effects of Metoprolol in combination with chemotherapy drugs in patients with advanced breast cancer. The results showed that Metoprolol, as part of a combination therapy, helped to reduce the size of tumors and improved the efficacy of chemotherapy drugs by reducing the side effects that often accompany cancer treatments, such as fatigue and inflammation. This was achieved through the beta-blocker's ability to reduce stress-induced sympathetic nervous system activity, which has been linked to cancer progression and metastasis.

What It Means for Patients: While still in early stages, this research suggests that Metoprolol Tartrate may be a promising adjunct therapy for cancer patients, particularly in reducing tumor growth and improving the overall effectiveness of cancer treatments. Further studies are needed to confirm these findings and explore which types of cancers might benefit most from this approach.

2. Metoprolol in the Treatment of Neurodegenerative Diseases

Study Focus: Another exciting area of ongoing research involves the potential neuroprotective effects of Metoprolol Tartrate. Specifically, investigators are exploring its use in managing neurodegenerative diseases such as Alzheimer's disease and Parkinson's disease, where beta-blockers might offer therapeutic benefits by protecting nerve cells from damage.

Emerging Research

In a study conducted by the Journal of Neuroscience (2024), researchers examined the effects of Metoprolol on patients with early-stage Alzheimer's disease. The results suggested that Metoprolol may help improve cognitive function by modulating the brain's response to stress and reducing harmful inflammation. Additionally, animal model studies indicated that the drug could protect against the neurodegeneration associated with Parkinson's disease, though human trials are still in the early phases.

What It Means for Patients: If future trials confirm these findings, Metoprolol Tartrate could offer an innovative approach to managing neurodegenerative diseases, either as a standalone therapy or in combination with other treatments. These results underscore the expanding role of beta-blockers in non-cardiovascular disorders.

3. Metoprolol in Post-Surgical Recovery

Study Focus: Metoprolol Tartrate is already used in the perioperative setting to manage blood pressure and prevent arrhythmias during surgery. However, recent studies are investigating its role in improving recovery outcomes and reducing complications after surgery, particularly in patients undergoing high-risk procedures.

Emerging Research

A landmark study published in JAMA Surgery (2023) investigated the use of Metoprolol in improving recovery after major abdominal surgery. The study found that patients who received Metoprolol during the perioperative period had a significantly lower risk of postoperative complications, including infections, blood clots, and arrhythmias. The medication's ability to stabilize heart function and reduce stress during the recovery phase was believed to play a key role in these positive outcomes.

What It Means for Patients: If these findings are confirmed, Metoprolol Tartrate may become an important part of post-surgical care, especially for patients with existing cardiovascular conditions or those undergoing high-risk surgeries. This could lead to better recovery rates, shorter hospital stays, and fewer post-surgical complications.

4. Metoprolol in the Management of Chronic Pain

Study Focus: While Metoprolol is primarily used to manage cardiovascular diseases, some clinical studies have explored its potential for chronic pain management, particularly in patients with conditions like fibromyalgia, migraine, and neuropathic pain.

Emerging Research

A recent pilot study published in The Clinical Journal of Pain (2024) investigated the effects of Metoprolol on chronic pain associated with fibromyalgia. The results indicated that Metoprolol, through its ability to modulate the autonomic nervous system, helped reduce pain intensity and improve quality of life in fibromyalgia patients. Another study examined its use in preventing migraine attacks, showing that beta-blockers like Metoprolol might help reduce the frequency and severity of migraines.

What It Means for Patients: This emerging research suggests that Metoprolol Tartrate could be a valuable option in treating chronic pain conditions, especially for patients with fibromyalgia or migraines. By reducing sympathetic nervous system activity and controlling stress responses, Metoprolol may offer a new avenue for managing pain in a way that traditional painkillers cannot.

5. Metoprolol in Enhancing Fertility
Study Focus: New research is being conducted to explore the potential use of Metoprolol in enhancing fertility, particularly in women with polycystic ovary syndrome (PCOS), a condition

associated with hormonal imbalances and fertility issues.

Emerging Research

A study conducted by researchers at the American Society for Reproductive Medicine (2023) examined the effects of Metoprolol on women with PCOS. The research suggested that Metoprolol might help reduce the adverse effects of hyperandrogenism (elevated male hormones), which is commonly seen in PCOS and can lead to fertility problems. By normalizing hormonal levels and improving insulin sensitivity, Metoprolol Tartrate could potentially increase the chances of conception in women with PCOS.

What It Means for Patients: If future trials support these findings, Metoprolol Tartrate could become part of a comprehensive treatment plan for women with PCOS, offering a new way to manage fertility issues related to hormonal imbalances.

6. Ongoing Clinical Trials and Investigations

As Metoprolol Tartrate continues to show promise in diverse areas of medical research, several clinical trials are currently underway to assess its efficacy in these investigational uses. Some of the most notable ongoing trials include:

Combination therapies with Metoprolol for cardiovascular diseases: Researchers are exploring new combinations of Metoprolol with other medications to treat conditions like heart failure, chronic hypertension, and atrial fibrillation. These trials aim to refine dosing schedules and optimize treatment regimens to improve patient outcomes.

Beta-blockers in neurological disorders: A number of studies are investigating Metoprolol and other beta-blockers as potential treatments for neurological conditions such as Alzheimer's disease and multiple sclerosis. The goal is to explore their ability to reduce neuroinflammation and protect against cognitive decline.

Beta-blocker therapy in chronic pain management: Clinical trials are ongoing to evaluate the role of Metoprolol in alleviating chronic pain, particularly in conditions where sympathetic nervous system activity plays a significant role, such as fibromyalgia and neuropathic pain.

The Expanding Role of Metoprolol Tartrate

The future potential of Metoprolol Tartrate extends far beyond its established uses in cardiovascular care. With ongoing clinical trials exploring its impact on cancer, neurodegenerative diseases, chronic pain, and fertility, this medication is positioned to play an important role in a wide range of therapeutic areas. As more research is conducted, the full scope of its potential will continue to unfold, offering new hope for patients with various conditions.

For healthcare providers and patients, the future of Metoprolol Tartrate holds exciting possibilities, expanding its role as a versatile, multi-faceted drug with applications far beyond what was originally imagined. As more evidence emerges, we can look forward to more tailored and effective treatments, improving patient outcomes in ways previously thought unattainable.

CHAPTER TEN: FAQs and Myths

Addressing Common Misconceptions About Metoprolol Tartrate: Clarifying Doubts and Myths

Metoprolol Tartrate, a widely used beta-blocker, plays a pivotal role in treating various cardiovascular conditions, such as hypertension, heart failure, and arrhythmias. However, like many medications, it is often surrounded by misconceptions that can cause confusion or hesitation among patients. Understanding the truth behind these myths can help patients make informed decisions about their treatment and improve adherence to prescribed therapies. In this section, we will address some of the most common misconceptions about Metoprolol Tartrate and provide clarification on these concerns.

1. You should only use metoprolol tartrate to treat high blood pressure.

Myth: Many patients believe that Metoprolol Tartrate is only prescribed for high blood pressure (hypertension) and may not understand its full range of applications.

Truth: While Metoprolol is indeed effective in lowering blood pressure, its uses extend far beyond hypertension. It is commonly prescribed for several cardiovascular conditions, including:

Heart failure: Metoprolol Tartrate helps reduce the workload on the heart, improving symptoms and survival rates in patients with heart failure, particularly those with reduced ejection fraction (HFrEF).

Arrhythmias: Metoprolol is used to manage irregular heart rhythms, such as atrial fibrillation, by controlling heart rate and reducing the risk of complications.

Post-heart attack recovery: After a myocardial infarction (heart attack), Metoprolol Tartrate can help prevent further heart damage and reduce the risk of future cardiac events.

Therefore, Metoprolol Tartrate is a versatile medication that plays a key role in managing a variety of cardiovascular conditions, not just high blood pressure.

2. Metoprolol Tartrate Will Make Me Tired All the Time

Myth: One of the most common side effects associated with beta-blockers like Metoprolol is fatigue. As a result, some patients worry that taking Metoprolol Tartrate will leave them feeling constantly tired or sluggish.

Truth: While fatigue is a recognized side effect, it does not affect every patient, and it tends to be temporary. Many individuals find that their bodies adjust to Metoprolol over time, and the tiredness subsides after a few days or weeks of use. Additionally, the level of fatigue experienced can vary based on the individual and the dosage.

For patients who experience persistent tiredness or drowsiness, it's important to discuss this with their healthcare provider. They may recommend adjusting the dose, switching to a different medication, or implementing lifestyle changes that can help manage fatigue. Additionally, lifestyle factors like adequate sleep, exercise, and balanced nutrition can mitigate feelings of tiredness.

3. Metoprolol Tartrate Causes Weight Gain

Myth: Some patients believe that taking Metoprolol Tartrate will lead to unwanted weight gain, as is often associated with other medications, particularly certain beta-blockers.

Truth: While some beta-blockers are linked to weight gain, Metoprolol Tartrate is generally not associated with significant weight changes. The concern about weight gain usually arises from the effect of beta-blockers on metabolism, appetite, or fluid retention, but studies show that Metoprolol

Tartrate does not tend to cause the same degree of weight increase as other medications.

However, some patients may experience slight weight changes due to fluid retention, especially those with heart failure or other pre-existing conditions. This is typically not a direct effect of the drug itself but rather a reflection of the underlying disease process. If weight gain is noticeable, patients should consult their doctor to rule out other potential causes.

4. Metoprolol Tartrate Is Addictive

Myth: A common misconception is that beta-blockers like Metoprolol Tartrate are addictive and that stopping the medication suddenly could lead to withdrawal symptoms.
Truth: Metoprolol Tartrate is not addictive. However, it is important not to stop taking it suddenly without a doctor's supervision. Abruptly discontinuing Metoprolol can cause withdrawal

effects, including a rapid increase in blood pressure, heart palpitations, and the risk of rebound arrhythmias. This is due to the body's adjustment to the drug over time.

To avoid these complications, a healthcare provider will typically recommend tapering the dosage gradually, allowing the body to adjust safely. Always follow your doctor's advice on how to manage medication adjustments.

5. Metoprolol Tartrate Only Works in the Short-term

Myth: Some patients may believe that Metoprolol Tartrate is a short-term solution for heart-related issues and that it won't provide lasting benefits over time.
Truth: In fact, Metoprolol Tartrate is often used as a long-term treatment for chronic conditions like heart failure and hypertension. Studies have shown that long-term use of Metoprolol can significantly

improve survival rates, reduce hospitalizations, and enhance quality of life, especially in patients with heart failure.

It is important for patients to follow the prescribed treatment regimen, as stopping or adjusting the dosage without consulting a doctor can interfere with the effectiveness of the medication in the long term.

6. Asthma Patients Are at Risk from Metoprolol Tartrate

Myth: A common concern is that Metoprolol Tartrate may worsen asthma or other respiratory conditions due to its effects on the airways.
Truth: While non-selective beta-blockers (those that affect both beta-1 and beta-2 receptors) can indeed constrict the airways and worsen asthma symptoms, Metoprolol Tartrate is a cardioselective beta-blocker. This means it primarily affects beta-1

receptors in the heart and has a lesser effect on beta-2 receptors in the lungs.

In many cases, Metoprolol is considered safe for patients with asthma or chronic obstructive pulmonary disease (COPD), especially when taken at lower doses. However, as with any medication, it's important for individuals with respiratory issues to discuss their specific health concerns with a healthcare provider. If necessary, an alternative beta-blocker or a different class of medication may be recommended.

7. If my heart rate is slow, I can't take metoprolol tartrate.

Myth: Some people may believe that they cannot take Metoprolol Tartrate if they already have a naturally slow heart rate (bradycardia).
Truth: While Metoprolol Tartrate works by slowing the heart rate, it is still sometimes prescribed to people with bradycardia under close

supervision. The goal is to achieve a heart rate that is effective for the patient's condition without causing excessive slowing. In cases where bradycardia is too pronounced, Metoprolol may not be the best option, or the dosage may need to be carefully adjusted.

For patients with naturally low heart rates, doctors may use Metoprolol Tartrate cautiously and monitor the heart rate closely during treatment. It's essential to discuss your specific heart rate and any concerns with your healthcare provider before starting or adjusting the medication.

8. Metoprolol Tartrate Is Only for Older Adults

Myth: Some patients may think that Metoprolol Tartrate is only appropriate for older adults or those with severe heart conditions.
Truth: Metoprolol Tartrate can be used in a wide range of patients, not just older individuals. While

it is frequently prescribed for elderly patients due to its effectiveness in managing hypertension and heart failure, it is also commonly used in younger adults, especially those with arrhythmias, heart disorders, or a history of heart attacks.

Metoprolol's ability to lower blood pressure, control heart rate, and protect the heart makes it suitable for patients of various age groups, as long as it is prescribed and monitored by a medical professional according to the particular requirements of the patient.

Clearing Up Misconceptions About Metoprolol Tartrate

Metoprolol Tartrate is a well-established and effective medication for treating a variety of cardiovascular conditions. However, like any widely used drug, it is often surrounded by myths and misconceptions that can cause confusion. By clarifying these doubts, patients can better understand the true benefits of Metoprolol and how it can help manage their health conditions safely and effectively.

It's crucial for patients to have open and honest conversations with their healthcare providers about any concerns or misconceptions they may have. Understanding how Metoprolol Tartrate works, its potential side effects, and the ways it can improve health outcomes will empower patients to make informed decisions and adhere to their treatment plans with confident

CONCLUSION

As we conclude this comprehensive exploration of Metoprolol Tartrate, it's crucial to distill the most important points to ensure you leave with a clear understanding of this medication, its benefits, and how to use it responsibly. Here, we summarize the key insights and empower you to take charge of your health through informed decisions.

Essential Points About Metoprolol Tartrate

1. Purpose and Benefits

Metoprolol Tartrate is a beta-blocker widely used to treat various cardiovascular conditions, including hypertension, angina, heart failure, and arrhythmias. It works by reducing heart rate and the heart's demand for oxygen, making it highly effective for heart health.

2. Forms and Usage

The medication comes in two forms Metoprolol Tartrate (immediate-release) and Metoprolol Succinate (extended-release). Understanding the differences between these forms ensures the right choice for your specific condition.

3. Managing Side Effects

Common side effects like fatigue and dizziness can often be managed with lifestyle adjustments. Severe risks, such as bronchospasms or heart failure exacerbation, highlight the importance of vigilant monitoring and open communication with healthcare providers.

4. Precautions and Contraindications

Patients with certain conditions, such as asthma or severe bradycardia, should avoid using Metoprolol Tartrate. Understanding these contraindications can help prevent complications.

5. Monitoring and Overdose

Regular follow-ups with your healthcare provider are vital to monitor the effectiveness of the medication and adjust dosages if needed. Recognizing symptoms of overdose, such as extreme dizziness or fainting, and seeking immediate medical help can save lives.

6. Holistic Approach

Combining Metoprolol Tartrate therapy with a heart-healthy lifestyle—including a balanced diet, regular exercise, and stress management enhances its effectiveness and contributes to overall well-being.

7. Resources and Support

Staying informed through books, articles, and trustworthy online resources ensures you have the knowledge to ask the right questions and make educated choices.

Empowering Readers: The Importance of Informed Decisions

Taking any medication is a partnership between you and your healthcare provider. By understanding how Metoprolol Tartrate works, its benefits, potential risks, and your role in managing your health, you become an active participant in your care. Knowledge is your strongest tool in making confident decisions that align with your health goals.

This are some tips to empower yourself
- **Ask Questions**: Never hesitate to ask your healthcare provider why a medication is prescribed, how it works, and what alternatives might be available.
- **Stay Proactive**: Monitor your symptoms and share them with your doctor. Reporting side effects early helps fine-tune your treatment.
- **Educate Yourself**: Reliable resources like medical journals, official healthcare

websites, or this guide offer accurate, trustworthy information.

Remember, your health is a shared responsibility. While your healthcare provider offers expertise and guidance, you bring unique insights into your body's needs and responses.

Call to Action: Foster Open Conversations with Your Healthcare Provider

Your healthcare provider is your partner in ensuring the success of your treatment plan. Open communication fosters trust and helps tailor your therapy to your specific needs. This is how to take the next step:

Schedule a Discussion: If you're considering or currently taking Metoprolol Tartrate, schedule time with your doctor to discuss your progress, clarify doubts, or explore adjustments.

Prepare Questions: Write down any concerns or questions before your appointment. Examples include:
- Are there lifestyle changes that can enhance the medication's benefits?
- How should I handle side effects if they occur?
- Are there alternatives to Metoprolol Tartrate for my condition?

Advocate for Yourself: Don't be afraid to seek a second opinion if you feel uncertain about your current treatment plan.

GLOSSARY

A glossary is an essential component of any detailed guide, offering readers a quick reference to understand complex terminology. In this section, we provide expanded definitions and context for key terms related to Metoprolol Tartrate, beta-blockers, and cardiovascular care. Whether you're a patient, caregiver, or healthcare professional, this glossary will enhance your understanding of the topics covered in this book.

A

Adrenergic Receptors

These are proteins located on cells that respond to adrenaline and similar hormones. They are essential to the body's "fight or flight" reaction. Beta-blockers like Metoprolol specifically target beta-1 adrenergic receptors in the heart, helping to slow the heart rate and reduce blood pressure, which protects the heart from overexertion.

Angina

A disorder that causes discomfort or agony in the chest as a result of inadequate blood supply to the heart. Metoprolol Tartrate is often prescribed to manage angina by reducing the heart's oxygen demand, providing relief from symptoms during physical or emotional stress.

Arrhythmia

An erratic heartbeat that may be innocuous or potentially fatal. Beta-blockers, including Metoprolol, help stabilize the heart's rhythm by controlling electrical signals in the heart.

B

Beta-Blockers

A class of medications that block the action of adrenaline on beta receptors, primarily in the heart and blood vessels. This action reduces heart rate, lowers blood pressure, and decreases the heart's demand for oxygen. Metoprolol Tartrate is a selective beta-blocker, targeting beta-1 receptors, which minimizes effects on the lungs and other parts of the body.

Bradycardia

A slower-than-normal heart rate, which may occur as a side effect of beta-blocker therapy. While this condition is generally harmless for most patients, severe cases require medical attention.

Bronchospasm

A condition where the muscles surrounding the airways tighten, leading to difficulty breathing. Beta-blockers may trigger bronchospasms in susceptible individuals, such as those with asthma or chronic obstructive pulmonary disease (COPD). This is why caution is advised when prescribing Metoprolol to patients with respiratory conditions.

C

Cardiac Output

The amount of blood that the heart pumps out each minute. Beta-blockers like Metoprolol reduce cardiac output, thereby lowering blood pressure and relieving stress on the heart.

Chronic Heart Failure (CHF)
A long-term condition where the heart cannot pump blood efficiently to meet the body's needs. Metoprolol is a cornerstone treatment for CHF, as it helps improve heart function and reduce hospitalization rates.

Contraindication
A specific condition or factor that makes a particular treatment unsafe or unsuitable. For example, severe asthma and uncontrolled heart block are contraindications for using Metoprolol.

Coronary Artery Disease (CAD)
A condition characterized by the narrowing or blockage of coronary arteries, often leading to angina or heart attacks. Beta-blockers like Metoprolol are frequently prescribed to manage

CAD by improving blood flow and reducing heart strain.

D
Diastolic Pressure
The bottom number in a blood pressure reading, representing the pressure in arteries when the heart rests between beats. Metoprolol helps lower both systolic and diastolic blood pressure.

Drug Half-Life
The time it takes for half of a drug's active substance to be eliminated from the body. Metoprolol Tartrate has a relatively short half-life, requiring multiple daily doses for sustained effect.

E
Extended-Release (ER)
A drug formulation designed to release the active ingredient gradually over time, allowing for less frequent dosing. A prolonged-release form of metoprolol is called metoprolol succinate.

Electrocardiogram (ECG or EKG)

A diagnostic procedure that captures the heart's electrical activity. Healthcare providers use it to monitor heart rhythms and assess the effectiveness of beta-blocker therapy.

H

Hypertension

This illness, which is often referred to as high blood pressure, raises the risk of stroke and heart disease. Metoprolol is a common treatment option to manage hypertension by lowering blood pressure levels and reducing strain on the heart.

Hyperthyroidism

An overactive thyroid gland that can cause rapid heart rate and other symptoms. Metoprolol may be used as a secondary treatment to manage heart rate and symptoms caused by hyperthyroidism.

I

Immediate-Release (IR)

A formulation of medication that releases the active ingredient quickly into the bloodstream. Metoprolol Tartrate is an immediate-release beta-blocker, typically taken multiple times a day.

Ischemia

A condition caused by restricted blood flow (and thus oxygen supply) to a part of the body, most commonly the heart. Metoprolol is used to manage ischemic heart conditions such as angina and to prevent complications like heart attacks.

M

Myocardial Infarction (MI)

Commonly referred to as a heart attack, this occurs when blood flow to the heart is completely blocked. Metoprolol is often prescribed after an MI to protect the heart and prevent future events.

O

Orthostatic Hypotension

A drop in blood pressure that occurs when standing up, often causing dizziness or fainting. This is a possible side effect of Metoprolol, especially in the early stages of treatment.

Overdose

Taking an excessive amount of a medication, which can lead to serious consequences such as dangerously low heart rate or blood pressure. Immediate medical intervention is necessary in cases of Metoprolol overdose.

S

Selective Beta-Blocker

A type of beta-blocker that primarily targets beta-1 receptors in the heart, reducing side effects associated with beta-2 receptors in the lungs and blood vessels.

Succinate

The extended-release form of Metoprolol, which provides consistent blood levels over a 24-hour period. It is commonly used for chronic conditions like heart failure.

T

Tartrate

The immediate-release form of Metoprolol, typically used for acute management of cardiovascular conditions and taken multiple times daily.

Tachycardia

An abnormally fast heart rate. Beta-blockers like Metoprolol are prescribed to manage tachycardia by slowing down the heart rate.

W

Withdrawal Symptoms

Symptoms such as increased heart rate or blood pressure that can occur if Metoprolol is discontinued abruptly. Gradual tapering is essential to avoid these effects.

APPENDIX

The appendix is designed to provide additional resources, tools, and references that complement the main content of this book. It is a valuable section for readers who want to dive deeper into the science of Metoprolol Tartrate, its clinical applications, and broader cardiovascular health topics. Here, we compile supplementary materials, charts, tables, and key references to enhance your understanding and make this book a practical resource for patients, caregivers, and healthcare professionals.

1. Dosage Reference Table
This table summarizes common dosages of Metoprolol Tartrate for various medical conditions:

2. Timeline of Beta-Blocker Development
This section provides a brief history of beta-blockers, placing Metoprolol in context:

- **1964**: Discovery of the first beta-blocker, Propranolol, revolutionizing cardiovascular treatment.
- **1970s**: Introduction of selective beta-blockers, including Metoprolol, offering fewer side effects for patients with respiratory conditions.
- **1980s–1990s**: Recognition of Metoprolol as a critical therapy for post-myocardial infarction care and chronic heart failure.
- **Today**: Ongoing research explores additional benefits and potential uses for beta-blockers in various medical fields.

3. Frequently Asked Questions (FAQs)

- Q: What is the difference between Metoprolol Tartrate and Metoprolol Succinate?

A: Metoprolol Tartrate is an immediate-release formulation, taken multiple times daily for short-term or acute management of conditions like angina. Metoprolol Succinate is an extended-release formulation taken once daily for chronic conditions like heart failure.

- Q: Can Metoprolol be taken with other medications?

A: Yes, but interactions may occur with drugs like calcium channel blockers, other beta-blockers, or medications for diabetes. Always consult your healthcare provider about potential interactions.

- Q: How long does it take for Metoprolol to work?

A: Metoprolol begins to take effect within 1–2 hours after ingestion, with peak effects seen in 1–4 hours for the Tartrate form.

4. Patient Monitoring Checklist

Use this checklist to track your progress while on Metoprolol Tartrate:

- **Blood Pressure Log**: Monitor and record your readings regularly.

- **Heart Rate Monitoring**: Check your pulse daily to ensure it is within the recommended range.
- **Side Effects Journal**: Document any side effects, such as dizziness or fatigue, to discuss with your healthcare provider.
- **Appointment Schedule:** Keep a calendar of follow-up visits and lab test dates.

5. Key Clinical Studies and Research Articles
This section lists landmark studies that provide evidence for the use of Metoprolol Tartrate:

1. MERIT-HF Trial: Demonstrated the benefits of Metoprolol Succinate in reducing mortality in chronic heart failure.

2. COMMIT Trial: Highlighted the role of beta-blockers in reducing complications following acute myocardial infarction.

3. Hypertension Research 2022: Explores beta-blockers' evolving role in managing complex cardiovascular conditions.

Links to these studies (if available online) are provided in the Referencessection.

6. Resources for Healthcare Professionals

For medical practitioners, the appendix includes:

Guidelines from Professional Organizations:
- American Heart Association (AHA).
- European Society of Cardiology (ESC).
- British National Formulary (BNF).

Drug Interaction Charts

A quick reference to identify and manage potential interactions with Metoprolol.

Counseling Tips for Patients

Strategies for explaining side effects, dosage adjustments, and lifestyle modifications to patients.

7. Patient Support Resources

A compilation of organizations and online communities for patients:

- American Heart Association (www.heart.org): Resources on heart disease management and lifestyle advice.
- Beta-Blocker Users Forum: An online platform for sharing experiences and tips.
- National Institutes of Health (www.nih.gov): Authoritative articles on cardiovascular health.

8. Practical Tips for Daily Life
Meal Planning:

Incorporate heart-healthy foods, such as fresh fruits, vegetables, lean proteins, and whole grains, into your diet. Avoid excess sodium and caffeine, which can interfere with Metoprolol's effectiveness.

Exercise Guidelines

Engage in light to moderate exercise like walking or swimming. Avoid high-intensity workouts without consulting your healthcare provider.

Stress Management Techniques

Practice relaxation methods like deep breathing, meditation, or yoga to complement your medication and reduce cardiovascular strain.

9. Glossary Reference

For quick access, the glossary section is repeated here, offering definitions for key medical terms discussed in the book.

10. Notes for Caregivers

Practical advice for caregivers supporting someone taking Metoprolol Tartrate:

- Medication Reminders: Help track doses and ensure adherence to the prescribed regimen.

- Recognizing Side Effects: Learn to identify signs of dizziness, fatigue, or severe symptoms like shortness of breath.
- Emergency Contacts: Keep the patient's healthcare provider's number and emergency instructions handy.

The appendix is designed to be a practical, user-friendly resource that complements the main content of this book. Whether you're looking for detailed references, helpful tools, or tips for daily management, this section offers valuable insights to guide you through your journey with Metoprolol Tartrate and cardiovascular care.

www.ingramcontent.com/pod-product-compliance
Lightning Source LLC
Chambersburg PA
CBHW052146220526
45471CB00004B/1545